Essentials of Internet Use in Nursing

Kristen S. Montgomery, PhD, RN is a Postdoctoral Research Fellow at the University of Michigan School of Nursing. She received her doctorate in nursing at the Frances Payne Bolton School of Nursing, Case Western Reserve University in Cleveland, Ohio. She earned her MSN from The University of Pennsylvania in Philadelphia, and her BSN from Oakland University. She is coeditor of the *Maternal Child Health Nursing Research Digest* and *Internet Resources for Nurses*, both of which received the *American Journal of Nursing* Book of the Year Award.

Joyce J. Fitzpatrick, PhD, MBA, RN, FAAN, is Elizabeth Brooks Ford Professor of Nursing, Frances Payne Bolton School of Nursing at Case Western Reserve University in Cleveland, Ohio, where she was Dean from 1982 through 1997. She earned her BSN at Georgetown University, her MS in Psychiatric-Mental Health Nursing at The Ohio State University, her PhD in Nursing at New York University, and an MBA from Case Western Reserve University in 1992. She has received 13 *American Journal of Nursing* Book of the Year Awards, the Midwest Nursing Research Society Award for Distinguished Contribution to Nursing Research, The Ohio State University Distinguished Alumna Award, the Sigma Theta Tau International Elizabeth McWilliams Miller Founders Award for Excellence in Nursing Research, as well as the New York University Division of Nursing Distinguished Alumna Award, and the American Nurses Foundation Distinguished Contribution to Nursing Science Award. Dr. Fitzpatrick is widely published in nursing and health care literature, having over 300 publications. She is coeditor of the *Annual Review of Nursing Research* series, now in its twentieth volume, and editor of the journals *Applied Nursing Research* and *Nursing Education Perspectives*. From 1997 to 1999, Dr. Fitzpatrick was President of the American Academy of Nursing.

Essentials of Internet Use in Nursing

Kristen S. Montgomery, PhD, RN
Joyce J. Fitzpatrick, PhD, RN, FAAN
Editors

 Springer Publishing Company

Copyright © 2002 by Springer Publishing Company, Inc.

Springer Publishing Company, Inc.
536 Broadway
New York, NY 10012-3955

Cover design by Joanne E. Honigman
Acquisitions Editor: Ruth Chasek
Production Editor: Pamela Lankas

02 03 04 05 06 / 5 4 3 2 1

Library of Congress Cataloging-in-Publication Data

Essentials of internet use in nursing / Kristen S. Montgomery, Joyce J. Fitzpatrick, editors.
    p. cm.
   Includes bibliographical references and index.
   ISBN 0-8261-1554-3
   1. Nurse—Computer network resources.   2. Internet.
3. Medical care—Computer network resources.

  RT50.5 .E85 2002
  025.06'61073—dc21   2002021043
                                      CIP

Printed in the United States of America by Capital City Press.

Contents

Part II: Education Applications

Part III: Other Applications

Preface

This book is meant to serve as a reference for nurses who use or are interested in using the Internet in their practice. It has been said repeatedly that the Internet is influencing health care and that Web sites grow in number each day. Although the number of health-related Web sites does indeed continue to grow, there is less information available on how to use these Web sites to improve professional nursing practice and, hence, improve patient care. Use of the Internet to improve patient care provides a vast amount of potential applications in virtually all areas that nurses practice. In several ways, *Essentials of Internet Use in Nursing* can be seen as a complementary text to two previously published Internet resources, Fitzpatrick and Montgomery (2000) *Internet Resources for Nurses* and Fitzpatrick, Romano, and Chasek (2001) *The Nurses' Guide to Consumer Health Web Sites*. Both of these texts highlight the best Internet sites for nurses and for nurses to recommend to patients. These books provide Internet content and *Essentials of Internet Use in Nursing* provides the process or "how-to" information on using the Internet to improve professional practice and patient care.

We believe that nurses function in a variety of overlapping roles. This belief has guided our development of this book as a comprehensive resource that addresses the main roles of professional nurses. The book is divided into three sections: the clinical setting, the education setting, and education applications to other pertinent settings. The clinical section addresses applications for professional nurses, system-wide issues, and patient care. The education section addresses distance education and continuing education. The other applications section addresses research, health policy, and interdisciplinary concerns.

We are hopeful that you will enjoy this book and will be successful in incorporating Internet use into your own professional practice.

REFERENCES

Fitzpatrick, J. J., & Montgomery, K. S. (Eds.). (2000). *Internet resources for nurses.* New York: Springer Publishing Co.

Fitzpatrick, J. J., Romano, C., & Chasek, R. (Eds). (2001). *The nurses' guide to consumer health Web sites.* New York: Springer Publishing Co.

Contributors

Patricia A. Abbott, PhD, RN, BC, FAAN
Assistant Professor and Coordinator
  of Graduate Programs in Nursing
  Informatics
School of Nursing
University of Maryland
Baltimore, MD

Julia W. Aucoin, DNS, RN
Consultant in Staff Development
  and Continuing Education
Tennessee Technological
  University
Cookville, TN

Jan V. R. Belcher, PhD, RN, CS
Associate Professor
College of Nursing and Health
Wright State University—
  Miami Valley
Dayton, OH

Cheryl Fisher, MSN, RN
Clinical Research Nurse
Heart, Lung, and Blood Institute
National Institutes of Health
Bethesda, MD

Maureen Gerrity, MS, RN
Nurse Clinician and Informatics
  Specialist
Neonatal Intensive Care Unit
The Johns Hopkins Hospital
Baltimore, MD

Janice L. Gibson, MS, RN
Senior Systems Analyst
Clinical Information Systems
University of Maryland Medical
  System
Baltimore, MD

Kimberly S. Glassman, MA, RN
Director of Care Management
New York University Medical Center
New York, NY

Carol Holdcraft, DNS, RN
Assistant Dean
College of Nursing and Health
Wright State University—
  Miami Valley
Dayton, OH

Michael Impollonia, MSN, RN, CNS
Manager, Nursing Recruitment and Retention
The Mount Sinai Hospital
New York, NY

Carole P. Jennings, PhD, RN
Assistant Professor
Coordinator-Nursing and Health Policy Graduate Program
School of Nursing
University of Maryland
Baltimore, MD

Trudy Johnson, MA, RN, CNAA
Director, Performance Improvement Services
New York-Presbyterian Hospital
New York, NY

Jane Koeckeritz, PhD, RN, C-ANP
Professor
School of Nursing
University of Northern Colorado
Greenley, CO

Mary L. McHugh, PhD, RN, BC, ARNP
Associate Professor
School of Nursing
University of Colorado Health Sciences Center
Denver, CO

Mary Etta C. Mills, ScD, RN, CNAA
Associate Professor and Director of Professional & Distributive Studies
School of Nursing
University of Maryland
Baltimore, MD

Georgia Narsavage, PhD, RN
Associate Professor and Director, Master's Programs
Frances Payne Bolton School of Nursing
Case Western Reserve University
Cleveland, OH

Jeanne M. Novotny, PhD, RN
Dean and Professor
School of Nursing
Fairfield University
Fairfield, CT

Carol Pullen, EdD, RN
Associate Professor and Assistant Dean for Rural Nursing Education
College of Nursing
University of Nebraska Medical Center
Omaha, NE

Hussein A. Tahan, MS, DNSc(c), RN, CNA
Director of Cardiovascular Nursing
New York-Presbyterian Hospital
New York, NY

Maria L. Vezina, EdD, RN
Director, Nursing Education and
    Recruitment
Department of Nursing
The Mount Sinai Hospital
New York, NY

**Patricia Hinton Walker, PhD,
    RN, FAAN**
AAN Senior Scholar In Residence
Center for Outcomes and
    Effectiveness Research
Agency for Healthcare Research
    and Quality and Professor
Rockville, MD
School of Nursing
University of Colorado Health
    Sciences Center
Denver, CO

Tami H. Wyatt, MSN, RN
Doctoral Student
School of Nursing
University of Virginia
Charlottesville, VA

Part I

Clinical Applications

Chapter 1

How to Find Information on the Internet

Kimberly S. Glassman

The Internet is a global communication network of computers with connections to telephone cables and satellite links (Gisby, 1997). Created as an electronic communication network for the U.S. Department of Defense in 1969, the Internet today allows millions of users to instantly have access to other people and information throughout the world (McCartney, 1999). There are five facilities available through the Internet: the World Wide Web, e-mail, newsgroups or discussion groups, file transfers, and telnet (Gisby, 1997). This chapter addresses the various ways nurses can use the Internet to enhance practice.

The World Wide Web is a vast directory of Internet addresses and "home pages" that allows users to more easily obtain the Internet information. Internet accounts are required in order to use the Internet. Some accounts can be obtained through providers such as universities, health care institutions, or libraries. These accounts often are free to employees and students. In most households, individuals purchase an Internet account through a commercial Internet service provider (ISP) such as America On-Line, Erols, and television cable companies. ISPs allow entry into the vast world of information through the use of a telephone line or cable connection and computer modem. Browsers, such as Netscape Navigator or Internet Explorer allow users to "browse" the Internet, and provide access to search engines, e-mail, and other Internet tools.

E-mail, or electronic mail, uses the Internet to send messages. E-mail is becoming a popular means of communication among the staff in many institutions, since it can communicate efficiently with any number of users simultaneously. Also, patients are using e-mail to communicate with health care providers, often making a visit unnecessary.

Newsgroups provide forums for users to discuss topics by text, rather than voice. A file transfer protocol (FTP) allows access to, and downloading of, pictures, graphics, text, and other documents from a remote computer. Telnet enables users to browse another's computer files (Gisby, 1997).

SEARCHING THE INTERNET

The first step in obtaining information on the Web is to conduct a search. The basic process of searching begins with selecting a topic, or a question to research. The user must then divide the topic or question into concepts, find the key words or phrases, and enter them into the search tool. Search tools are a major feature of the Internet that nurses need to master in order to obtain pertinent clinical information. Common search tools are AltaVista, Lycos, and Yahoo. The search engine is the component of the search tool that determines how it searches its database (Sparks & Rizzolo, 1998). The user types in a word or phrase, and the engine obtains the Web site information from its database, using a specific set of rules and logic. The user is then presented with a varying number of Web sites to review. Some broad term searches, such as "pressure ulcer" or "wound care," can yield thousands of Web sites that reference combinations of products for purchase, educational programs, articles, and guidelines. However, Web search engines often do not provide a ranking of the results, leaving the user to sort through vast amounts of useless information, or refine the search. Finding the appropriate clinical information to support practice requires skill in evaluating Web sites.

Evaluating the Web sites obtained from a search for clinical practice relevance is not an easy task. Because the World Wide Web has no oversight, it offers individuals the ability to post a Web page with personal information. Within many health-related Internet searches, there are many Web sites that contain unsubstantiated information and personal experiences of the author. While these sites may be useful to consumers who share an illness or for clinicians to "take the pulse" of their patient population, this information is often not based on scientific fact, and should not be used for medical or health advice. The vast amount of information on the Internet makes it imperative for nurses to be able to critically appraise medical or health information obtained through the Web. The Health on the Net Foundation offers a code of conduct to guide Web developers and clinicians in evaluating health-related Web sites. This code is available at *http://www.hon.ch/ HONcode/Conduct.html.*

World Wide Web site names and addresses are called "uniform resource locators" or URLs. URLs that end in the suffixes ".gov" or ".org" generally indicate sites that are government or professional society-sponsored. These sites are helpful for evidence-based information that can be applied to practice settings. The Internet makes extensive information searches more efficient by gathering the Web sites that include the search terms indicated by the user. The user can then refine the search to limit the sites retrieved to a more manageable amount. Many Web sites and reference libraries offer searching tips on their own Web sites. For a more academic approach to searching, the University of Florida Health Sciences Library provides a tutorial on searches at *http://www.library.health.ufl.edu/pubmed/pubmed2/ overview.html.* Medical librarians are considered to be experts in evaluating Web sites for consumer health information. Many academic medical center libraries, as well as public libraries, offer workshops for consumers to evaluate Web sites. The Patient and Family Resource Center at New York University Medical Center offers an "Ask a Librarian" feature to assist providers and consumers in obtaining health information on the Web. A medical librarian can offer an efficient service to clinicians, who may not have the time to do the Web search themselves, but can scan the written information or Web sites retrieved by the library service. The NYU site can be accessed at *http://library.med. nyu.edu/HCC/.*

In addition, there are many journal articles that provide simple tips to nurses on how to conduct an Internet search using specific topic examples (Blackburn, 1999; Gomez, DuBois, & King, 1998), and more extensive explanation of various search tools (Sparks & Rizzolo, 1998).

USES OF THE INTERNET IN PRACTICE

Bischoff and Kelley (1999) describe an emerging role for nurses as information brokers. Consumers and patients often come to health appointments armed with information from the Internet. Nurses are now required to respond to patients who often have more depth of knowledge about their diseases and conditions, and who have more sophisticated questions about their health. Nurses are in a key position to assist patients in the use and evaluation of Internet content, and therefore must become expert Internet consumers. (Please see Fitzpatrick, Romano, and Chasek [2001] for additional information on consumer health Web sites).

Keeping abreast of one's practice is time consuming, yet can be handled efficiently with Internet tools. Subscriptions to free Internet services such as the Morbidity and Mortality Weekly Reports, Medscape's Medpulse, and various discussion lists or listservs from professional nursing and specialty groups are ways to receive information via e-mail on a regular basis (Bischoff & Kelley, 1999). Discussion lists provide an electronic communication link to nurses with shared interests. Those listservs that offer a "digest" version that provides all of the daily messages in one e-mail limits the number of e-mails received each day. McCartney (1999) provides some strategies for nurses wishing to join a listserv, including discussion list "netiquette," maintaining confidentiality, and posing questions to the discussion group.

Through an affiliation with universities and health facilities, some nurses can obtain free subscriptions to journal services such as Ingenta that e-mail the table of contents of a variety of professional nursing journals or search the literature for recently published articles based on a variety of user-defined search terms (*http://www.ingenta.com*). Several professional nursing organizations have published handy reference guides for searching the Internet and evaluating the information received. In particular, AORN Journal (Drake, C., 1999, 2000), and the Journal of Emergency Nursing (Bradley, 1999; Vaughn & Bradley, 1999) have regular information columns for nurses using the Internet to obtain information to support their clinical practice.

The Internet provides a global perspective to nurses interested in exploring practice in other parts of the world. In a review of selected Web sites for neonatal nurses, the author describes an international discussion forum called Neonatal Talk (Blackburn, 1999). Here nurses from around the world can share practice experience on specific issues concerning the care of neonates. Blackburn (1999) also notes other sites of interest to neonatal nurses as an example of the richness of resources that can be obtained via the Internet. These resources include subscriptions to professional journals in electronic form, Web sites from academic medical centers that provide published practice guidelines, the Cochrane Collaboration for evidence-based practice reviews, and Web sites that provide continuing education for neonatal nurses.

EVIDENCE-BASED PRACTICE

Nurses have shown a growing interest in pursuing evidence-based practice. An easy way to begin using clinical evidence to support practice is to incorporate the many practice guidelines developed by government agencies and professional societies into institutional standards of care. Locating these guidelines can be done very easily over the Internet.

The National Guideline Clearinghouse (NGC) is a comprehensive database of evidence-based clinical practice guidelines and related documents produced by the Agency for Healthcare Research and Quality (AHRQ) (formerly the Agency for Health Care Policy and Research [AHCPR]), in partnership with the American Medical Association (AMA) and the American Association of Health Plans (AAHP). The NGC mission is to provide physicians, nurses, and other health professionals, an accessible mechanism for obtaining objective, detailed information on clinical practice guidelines and to further their dissemination, implementation, and use. Key components of NGC include: structured abstracts (summaries) about the guideline and its development; a utility for comparing attributes of two or more guidelines in a side-by-side comparison; syntheses of guidelines covering similar topics, highlighting areas of similarity and difference; links to full-text guidelines, where available, and/or ordering information for print copies; an electronic forum, NGC-L, for exchanging information on clinical practice guidelines and their development, implementation, and use; and annotated bibliographies on guideline development methodology, implementation, and use. The Web site can be accessed at: *http://www.guideline.gov/body_home.asp*. In addition, professional society Web sites reference their guidelines, and offer links to other sites that may be of interest to the user.

STRENGTHS AND WEAKNESSES OF USING THE INTERNET TO SUPPORT PRACTICE

The strengths of using the Internet to support practice are 1) access to vast amounts of information, and 2) efficiency. The explosion of

Web-based information provides ready access to volumes of clinically appropriate information. This strength, however, also serves as a major weakness, in that reviewing the sites/articles retrieved is often more time-consuming than busy clinicians can manage. The "bookmark" or "favorites" feature of many browsers can serve to facilitate immediate access to preferred Web sites, particularly government or professional society Web sites that update their content on a regular basis. (Please see Fitzpatrick and Montgomery [2000] for additional information on Web sites for professional nurses).

Some Web sites offer a variety of services on one site, an advantage for busy clinicians. Medscape, for example, is a free, commercial Web site that offers a vast collection of full-text clinical articles enhanced with keyword searches, graphics, and annotated links to Internet resources such as MEDLINE and full-text articles. Medscape provides daily updates specific to the nursing community via their homepage, including conference proceedings, and new technologies and treatments that are in the general news and thus may be of interest to patients and consumers. Nurses can receive a free weekly newsletter with summaries of health-related news from the prior week. Medscape also provides consumer information, and patient education handouts on various diseases and conditions.

PRACTICAL CONSIDERATIONS AND RESOURCES NEEDED

There are several considerations to using the Internet to support nursing practice. The availability of appropriate equipment and the costs of equipment maintenance must be considered. Most facilities have some computer hardware available, but it is not always convenient or configured for clinicians to use on the nursing units. Some older computers may not be able to download material with large files such as images, photographs, or other types of graphics. In these instances health facilities and nursing departments might consider partnering with a local public library and explore ways to use other resources to obtain specific information for use in patient care. Likewise, medical libraries may have a consumer division that can provide modest support to local clinicians.

For those areas where computer resources are readily available, clinician time is often the obstacle to obtaining pertinent clinical information. In this case, the development of "knowledge brokers" among interested staff may facilitate information exchange. Interested staff could become expert in searching the Internet, and obtain the information for their colleagues. An effective division of labor could include those nurses who are expert searchers and gatherers of information for others who agree to read and interpret the volumes of information obtained. At some academic medical centers, where access to academic resources is present, teams of clinicians work together to develop patient care standards. The clinical experts define the search terms, interested nurses conduct the search on the Internet and on library databases to obtain the articles or practice guidelines, and the team participates in the reading, evaluation, and development of the practice standard.

An academic-agency collaborative model was used to develop a workshop to enhance women's-health nurse practitioners' use of Internet resources (Carlton & Kelsey, 1997). A nurse practitioner provided the clinical specialty content for the workshop, while the academic partner provided the technology integration and electronic linking of user to resources. Through such partnering, and a positive response from attendees, a series of workshops was developed to continue to promote such expertise among the agency's advanced practice and staff nurses. Academic-agency partnerships have flourished in other areas as well. At NYU Medical Center and New York University's Division of Nursing, a pilot program was created to teach staff nurses and nursing students how to do online searches of the literature and the Internet. The medical librarians from the academic medical centers of Mount Sinai NYU Health, in collaboration with the Health Sciences librarians from NYU, developed a Web-based tutorial that provides a self-learning module to improve nurses' ability to use Internet resources. This three-part module addresses searching the literature, research utilization and evidence-based practice, and searching the Web. With this training, it is expected that nurses will develop the skills necessary to conduct such searches more efficiently on specific topics that will help them improve care.

Although computer use among nurses in the workplace is gradually becoming the norm, the effectiveness of its use to improve patient care is open to question. In a recent survey of computer use among nurse practitioners working in public, private, and HMO work sites ($n = 104$), 94% indicated that they used computers in their work (Dumas, Dietz, & Connolly, 2001). Although Internet searches were perceived by the nurse practitioners to be one of the most useful applications for improving care, less than half of those surveyed used their computers for Internet searches. The reasons cited for underutilization of computer technology were lack of availability of equipment and hardware that was dedicated for other uses such as patient billing or word processing.

FUTURE DEVELOPMENTS

The need for readily available clinical information continues to grow. Increasingly, networked computers can be found in many nurses' work settings. Access to the Internet is becoming more prevalent, and the use of handheld devices with drug reference software and other clinical information is already available for some clinician's use.

SUMMARY

The Internet offers a rich opportunity for nurses to gain knowledge and information to enhance clinical practice. Internet access is available in many hospitals and clinics, and in many homes. The challenge for practicing nurses is no longer accessibility, but rather how to sift through the copious material to quickly find the best information to support practice. Internet tools such as listservs, news groups, and topic searches conducted with expertise can help nurses manage current information that can be used to support patient care.

WEB SITE RECAP

Health on the Net (HON) Foundation Code of Conduct
http://www.hon.ch/HONcode/Conduct.html

Ingenta
http://www.ingenta.com

National Guideline Clearinghouse
http://www.guideline.gov/body_home.asp

Patient and Family Resource Center
http://library.med.nyu.edu/HCC/

University of Florida Health Sciences Library
http://www.library.health.ufl.edu/pubmed/pubmed2/overview.html

REFERENCES

Bischoff, W. R., & Kelley, S. J. (1999). 21st century house call: The Internet and the World Wide Web. *Holistic Nursing Practice, 13*(4), 42–50.

Blackburn, S. (1999). Internet resources for neonatal nurses. *Journal of Perinatal Neonatal Nursing, 12*(4), 41–52.

Bradley, V. (1999). WWW: Something for everyone. *Journal of Emergency Nursing, 25*, 139–141.

Carlton, K. H., & Kelsey, B. (1997). Partnerships for health care practice information. *Computers in Nursing, 15*, 117–127.

Drake, C. (1999). Internet resources for pressure ulcers prevention and treatment. *AORN Journal, 70*, 502–503.

Drake, C. (2000). Finding Internet resources about geriatric issues. *AORN Journal, 72*, 300–301.

Dumas, J., Dietz, E. O., & Connolly, P. M. (2001). Nurse practitioner use of computer technologies in practice. *Computers in Nursing, 19*, 34–40.

Fitzpatrick, J. J., & Montgomery, K. S. (Eds.) (2000). *Internet resources for nurses.* New York: Springer Publishing Co.

Fitzpatrick, J. J., Romano, C., & Chasek, R. (Eds.) (2001). *The nurses' guide to consumer health Web sites.* New York: Springer Publishing Co.

Gisby, J. (1997). Nursing and the Internet. *Nursing Standard, 11*(51), 60.

Gomez, E. G., DuBois, K., & King, C. R. (1998). Improving oncology nursing practice through understanding and exploring the Internet. *Oncology Nursing Forum, 25*(10 Suppl.), 4–10.

McCartney, P. R. (1999). Internet communication and discussion lists for perinatal nurses. *Journal of Perinatal Neonatal Nursing, 12*, 26–40.

Sparks, S. M., & Rizzolo, M. A. (1998). World Wide Web search tools. *Image: The Journal of Nursing Scholarship, 30*, 167–171.

Vaughn, M., & Bradley, V. (1999). Bookmarks for trauma Web resources. *Journal of Emergency Nursing, 25*, 538–540.

Chapter 2

Using the Internet in Clinical Settings: An Overview

Mary L. McHugh

T he great power of nurses comes from the specialized knowledge of the nurse. This knowledge is the basis of the lifesaving and health preserving services nurses provide to patients, and the reason the services of professional nurses are in such great demand in the early 21st century. All professional nurses in America have undergone a rigorous and scientifically based educational program. Each state further tests that knowledge before issuing a license to practice nursing. An important part of the knowledge imparted during the educational process is the understanding that the knowledge acquisition process must never stop. Of course, the nursing student is also provided with extensive knowledge about how to search the professional literature so that the process of lifelong continuing education is sustained. The Internet has become an important tool for nurses to use in advancing their knowledge. An incredible wealth of professional, peer-reviewed information is available through the Internet if one knows how to perform a search. In this chapter, uses of the Internet to support and expand nursing knowledge will be explored.

The benefits of having the Internet available to all nurses at their clinical sites fall generally into one of three categories: obtaining information related to the nurse's job and job duties, developing and expanding the nurse's network of contacts with professional colleagues, and using the Internet to improve professional practice within the institution. The first two categories are relatively obvious. The last category involves the nursing department as a whole. It addresses such areas as obtaining information and support for advancing the professional practice model in the hospital, advancing knowledge related to improving quality in the institution, and other department-wide information and communication issues.

Before nurses use information from the Internet in their clinical work, it is important to be sure the information is evaluated for both currency and credibility. In a review of over 30 papers that evaluated the quality of health information on the Internet, the majority of reviewers concluded that the information was not evidence based (Eysenbach, Yihune, Lampe, Cross, & Brickley, 1998). One serious problem with the Internet is that information often lacks a date of entry or update. Thus, one might be looking at information on a site that was sponsored by a well-known source, but if the date the information was entered is not listed, the accuracy of the information becomes a question. All the health care disciplines constantly conduct research to increase and improve their clinical knowledge. Thus, the date the information was entered is important. If one was looking at a site pertaining to current knee replacement techniques, it would matter if the site was one year old or if it was 5 years old. Science is changing so fast that information provided in a 5-year-old site would be outdated.

The most important question a nurse should ask about information acquired from the Internet is "How credible is this site?" In addition to all the excellent sites on the Internet that carry useful and reliable information, the nurse must be aware that there is also much misinformation on the Web. Anyone with the money to buy space and the skill to use a simple Web page construction program can put almost anything he or she wishes on the Internet. And seldom does a crackpot label his or her information with warning signs! Where the Internet is concerned, it is truly "buyer beware." The question therefore arises "How does the nurse decide whether or not to use the information found on a particular Web site?" There are several criteria by which the nurse should evaluate the credibility of any Web site that provides information on matters of clinical interest.

SELECTING CREDIBLE SITES

Site Sponsorship

The first and most important criterion relates to sponsorship of the site. The site's information can generally be relied upon if the site sponsor is credible (e.g., a known college or university medical center, scientific research institute or foundation, or association for a particular disease, such as the American Cancer Society). Some very famous clinicians also have sponsored their own sites. If the physician or nurse who put the information on the Internet is well known to the searcher, then the Web owner's reputation as a professional is probably also well known. The more likely scenario, however, is that the searcher does not know the Web owner. Then one might have a bit of work to do to ascertain the legitimacy of the information. Unfortunately, possession of a nursing or medical degree does not offer a guarantee that the owner will not become involved in a campaign to promote an untested therapeutic modality. When a professional allows his or her passion for a modality—often a nontraditional treatment modality—to overwhelm his or her scientific training, that professional may end up endorsing something that has no scientific validity. Even more unfortunate, some credentialed health care professionals become engaged in a business endeavor and use their credentials to promote products and treatment modalities that are questionable at best. However, there are some questions the nurse can ask to select the most credible sites to use.

The first three questions to ask are: (1) "Is the owner of this site using the site to sell some treatment or product rather than to simply give information?" (2) "Does the clinician who owns the Web site hold a position in a credible clinical agency?" And (3) "Is the site actually sponsored by that clinical agency?" Anyone who has gone into business for him/herself and is selling medical treatments, medications, or remedies on the Internet has a profit motive. The desire to make money can lead even professional health care providers to engage in questionable practices. Some physicians and nurses may have their own agendas that may not be congruent with the standards of scientific, evidence-based practice. Some might be selling worthless treatments and products to make money. Some might have become enamored with a treatment modality or product that they truly believe to be beneficial, yet the benefits have never been supported by research. Some might merely be greedy and want money regardless of the benefits or harm. Therefore, the mere fact that the Web site sponsor is a physician, nurse, physical therapist, or any other type of health care provider does not necessarily mean that the information on the site is either credible or safe.

A credible person who wishes to offer important health information on a Web site will make it clear exactly what information is being offered and what products are being sold. He or she will not use pressure tactics to coerce someone into ordering products he/she does not need. To assess credibility, phone the organization listed as the clinician's employer and ascertain if the person listed does indeed work in the position indicated at the agency. If not, has she/he recently moved to another job or position inside or external to the listed agency? If the clinical agency has never heard of the person that listed the agency as an employer, none of the site information should be trusted.

Site Ownership

The second criterion is to be sure that the site is actually owned by the person or agency it seems to represent. If a known clinical agency, scientific foundation, or disease association sponsors the site, credibility still needs to be assessed to ensure the site is not a "copycat" site. Web addresses have not existed for very many years and a Web address is purchased—not owned by virtue of a copyright or brand name. In 1992, there were only about 50–100 actual sites on the Internet—today there are over a billion sites. In the early years of the Internet, many established agencies were not even thinking about the Internet, much less purchasing the Web address closest to their name. At that time, some individuals purchased Web addresses that clearly fit the names of well-known companies. These high-profile names were "purchased" by people who either wanted to force the well-known company to pay a highly inflated price to buy its own name, or who wanted their site viewed by millions of people.

Today, there is a small war going on in the Internet business between nationally or internationally known organizations and unscrupulous but unknown persons who bought the companies' names to use as part of their Web addresses. The case today is, however, that simply because the nurse types in *www.well-known-name.com*, there is no automatic guarantee that the site reached will actually be owned by the credible and well-known agency. Some ways to be sure the site reached is actually owned by the desired agency is to check to be sure the agency's address is listed as a contact on the site. Search for other cues, such as a known phone number, perhaps a known executive officer or famous physician, or other cues that the site is actually owned by the desired agency.

Peer Reviewed Nature of Information

The third criterion for using information from the Web is that other experts in the field should have validated the information. As previously noted, anyone with the means and Web page building skills can put up papers they have written. Materials placed on the Web by credible foundations, universities, and health care organizations will have been carefully reviewed by experts prior to placement on the Web. The nurse may, however, find a variety of full-text papers that appear to be highly professional and published by credible clinicians or researchers.

Before using what is apparently a scientific paper, the nurse should be sure the paper was published by a reputable journal or reviewed by scientists and clinicians at a well-known university or clinical facility. Perhaps the greatest importance of professional journals is that all the papers they publish are "peer reviewed" before they are published. That is, most such journals subject every paper they publish to careful scrutiny by known experts in the field *before* allowing it to be published. The peer review process is the most important service offered by scientific and clinical health discipline journals. This means that the author is not publishing his or her own unfounded, untested personal opinions as scientific knowledge. Other scientists and clinical experts review the paper before it is published. Papers that contain claims about diagnostic methods, medications, or treatments that are outlandish or not supported by evidence or validated by known experts in the field are simply rejected by the reviewers and do not appear in the journal. Thus, it behooves the nurse to use only full-text papers that have been published by respectable health care journals. The fact that "Jane Doe" has placed on the Web a beautifully word-processed paper that carries the appearance of a professional journal article does not mean that it is credible. Unless the paper is a full-text article from a peer-reviewed journal, the nurse should ignore it.

Although nurses themselves struggle with determining whether or not a site's information is trustworthy, nurses must also advise their patients. A variety of studies have addressed patient use of the Internet (D'Alessandro & Dosa, 2001; Hejlesen et al., 1993; Goldberg, Morales, Gottlieb, Meador, & Safran, 2001; Abidi, Han, & Abidi, 2001; Smart & Burling, 2001). Although these studies address patient willingness and ability to use the Internet for health care purposes, none addressed the problem of teaching patients how to discriminate credible from worthless or even misleading sites. Nurses and physicians need guidelines for site selection. The preceding information is offered to help professionals begin the process of developing guidelines for Internet site selection for use in acquiring credible information about issues in health care. Please see Fitzpatrick and Montgomery (2000) and Fitzpatrick, Romano, and Chasek (2001) for additional information.

CLINICAL KNOWLEDGE ACQUISITION

There are an incredible number of sites on the Internet that provide nursing information. The quality of that information ranges from low to very high, and the depth of the information ranges from superficial to advanced. If the hospital's library subscribes to services like OVID that offer literature search capabilities and provide online access to full text articles, the Internet can be a very rich source of professional information. Other subscription sites can support orientation of new nurses and can provide fully accredited continuing education. Hospital educators can also create internally owned Web sites where employees can fulfill annual recertification for topics such as fire safety, blood-borne pathogens, hazardous materials handling, and the like.

Clinical educators' jobs have become extremely demanding. As these professionals seek to increase their productivity, more and more they are seeking technology that allows newly hired nurses to obtain a great deal of their orientation information from materials the clinical educator has placed on a hospital-owned Web site. Even without access to the extensive professional information available through professional libraries, there is a wealth of free information about clinical nursing on the Internet. Areas most useful to nurses include sources of knowledge about medications, peer reviewed professional papers that address clinical nursing problems, and online continuing education (including new nurse orientation support).

Medication Information

One type of knowledge that nurses frequently need quickly and accurately is information about medications their patients have taken or need to take. The number of medications available today is so large that no nurse can possibly know all of them, much less their primary effects, side effects, contraindications, and interactions with other medications. The rule all nurses were taught in school is, "Look up any unfamiliar medication before administering it to a patient." What the nurses were not taught was how to find the time to conduct such searches in a busy patient care setting.

One can only guess how many medication errors have been made because the nurse did not have the time to stop and look up an unfamiliar medication in the *Physician's Desk Reference* (PDR). Although the PDR and perhaps a formulary of some sort are likely to be available in most clinical settings in which nurses practice, the number of medication errors made in hospitals suggests that nurses do not use them as much as they should. The time consumed and inconvenience of using paper references may be a significant barrier to their use in clinical settings. Fortunately, reference books are not the only resources available today for medication searching.

It seems reasonable that if a computer search were to display the requisite information in a matter of seconds, more nurses would check out unfamiliar medications before administering them to patients. Computer searches can be extremely fast in comparison with searching for the unit's PDR—and then searching through the PDR. This is especially true if the nurse only knows the approximate spelling of the medication. Computer programs can easily "search for all similar" spellings, thus rapidly finding all the medications with similar names so the nurse can more quickly find the correct medication. In addition, the computer can search more rapidly than any human through 2,000 to 3,000 pages of a medication information database to find the desired medication listing. Several pharmaceutical companies have developed CD-ROM products that contain much information about medications, but few clinical units have those available. Lack of availability is a common problem because these products must be updated at least yearly because new medications are introduced frequently. The Internet contains a large number of sites that provide information on various medications. Internet sites can be updated daily and thus can be kept more current than fixed-information products such as books or CD-ROMs. Please see Montgomery and Uysal (2000) and Montgomery (2001) for additional medication information.

There are several possibilities available to nurses who wish to use the Internet to search for information on a particular medication. First, the hospital, clinic, or other agency may contract with a pharmaceutical company to offer their medication search program to all the units in the organization. Pharmaceutical companies typically update these products regularly and can provide access through its Internet site. If the pharmaceutical company wishes to restrict access to professionals or paid subscribers, password protections are available. It is also technically possible for access to be restricted to previously identified computers. In that way, no password is needed. Computers that can access the site have special programs installed that automatically identify the hospital computer as a legitimate user. The site can be bookmarked for instantaneous future access by the nurse.

Second, there are quite a number of search engines and sites on the Internet that can be used to find information on medications and any number of other topics. AltaVista.com is a search engine that was designed by Digital Corporation for scientists and professionals who wanted to find sites that gave them specific, high-quality professional information. It still does a very good job at that task. In addition, if the user needs to search for particular photos, graphics, or other images, AltaVista.com has a special image-search capability. Many other search engines too often do a better job of finding advertising than they do at finding professional information sites.

One site stands out as an excellent source of professional health care information. The National Library of Medicine (NLM) (*http://www.nlm.nih.gov*) offers many sources of information that are useful to the nurse seeking professional and scientific health care content. First and foremost, the NLM sponsors Medline. Medline is the online version of the old paper-based Index Medicus, which indexes published articles in over 4,300 professional health care journals. Additionally, Medline offers access to some health conference proceedings, reports of clinical trials, and LOCATOR*plus*, which catalogs books, journals, and audiovisual materials in the NLM collection. Professional research papers dealing with almost any clinical question on which nurses might seek clinical or research information are listed—often with the abstracts—on Medline.

The NLM site can be searched for information on a variety of medications, including new cancer medication trials. In addition, some pharmaceutical companies provide information about their products online. A quick way to find out about a particular medication is to go to the site of the company that produces the medication and see what information is available. For example, if the reader goes to the AltaVista site and types "Novartis Pharmaceuticals" into the search text line, one of the first ten sites listed is "Novartis Pharmaceuticals Corporation," which is the listing for the home page of the company. One of the hyperlinks on the site is labeled "products." Clicking on the "products" link brings up a list of the company's products, each of which is a hyperlink to a page about that medication.

Another way to search for pharmaceutical company sites when you do not know the correct spelling of the company name is to go to the Yahoo! site that provides a list of pharmaceutical companies (*http:// cf.us.biz.yahoo.com/p/_health-majrrx.html*). Clicking on the company will not take the nurse to the company home page. It will provide a business analysis of the company which may not be of help. However, the Yahoo! site is useful because the correct spelling of the names of many pharmaceutical companies can be obtained from the site and then entered into AltaVista (or another search engine) to search for the company's home page. Many of those pharmaceutical company sites provide a great deal of information about their products.

Clinical Information Search

Disease and treatment information. From time to time, most nurses will have a patient with a comorbidity diagnosis that he or she is not familiar with. The condition may be uncommon and the references on the unit may not provide adequate information. Fortunately, a very large number of medical conditions have sites on the Internet. In many cases, the sites were developed as self-help sites for people suffering from the unusual condition. These sites will be especially helpful to the nurses because they typically provide a lot of basic information about the condition and its treatment. The sites usually are written in simple language, often offer phone numbers of experts and self-help groups, and may provide references to other sites and further literature about the condition. Often the sites also will provide information on diagnostic criteria and treatment regimens. These may be especially helpful because the nurse unfamiliar with a condition will usually not know what kind of care is indicated.

For example, an AltaVista search on *sarcoidosis* found 25,320 listings. Obviously, searching so many sites would not be feasible, but fortunately the search engine has programming that brings up the most appropriate sites in the first few pages. The first site for Sarcoidosis was the American Lung Association, which is, of course, a highly credible source of information. This site begins by defining the disease, describing its symptoms, its usual course, its complications, and its treatment. The second site listed was a patient-centered, self-help site at: *http://www.worldsarcsociety.com/*. The World Sarcoidosis Society, based in Canada, is open to anyone who wishes to sign in. Among the many links in the site are a sarcoidosis newsletter, information for parents of children with sarcoidosis, and chat facilities for someone who just wants to talk to another sarcoidosis sufferer. The site has links to several physicians who treat the disorder and can be contacted for clinical advice. Other links are to American researchers who are conducting medication trials and other studies on the disease. Generally, finding the names of these researchers will help the nurse identify relevant literature on Medline. The third site listed is the sarcoidosis page in the Arthritis Foundation Web page. Although there are undoubtedly some sites that should not be used because of nonprofessional or untested medical information, the nurse can easily identify credible sites by the sponsor of the site.

Instructions and other information for patients. More and more hospitals and clinics have their own servers and can support locally designed information sites. These sites may require passwords to access. Many, however, are public. Just as many hospitals have long supported a local cable TV channel in their hospital that provided health programming, many hospitals are now supporting Internet sites that provide a variety of patient information.

One suggestion has been to place discharge instructions to patients and families on the Internet. Sheets with handwritten instructions that are typically given to patients often get lost or damaged in the bustle of trying to get home. For patients with an e-mail address, it would be very easy to both e-mail and print out the instructions. Since most outpatient surgery instructions follow a few standard rules, some of those kinds of instructions could also be made available on the Internet. In fact, many of the instructions sent home with outpatient procedure patients have more to do with the type of anesthesia provided than with the actual surgical procedure. Those could easily be made available on the Internet.

For example, in the field of orthopedic surgery alone there are a large number of patients who have procedures with fairly long recovery and therapy periods. Such commonly performed procedures as total knee and anterior cruciate ligament (ACL) replacements, hip replacements, arthroscopy of various joints, and the like, will require the patient to follow self-care and physical therapy regimens for several weeks or more after surgery. Internet sites could provide information on the typical course of recovery, indications of complications to watch for, how to respond if complications occur, and self care advice. Such information might not only save many unnecessary phone calls to the physician's office, they also might help the patient remember to perform the self-care activities recommended by the surgeon.

In addition, there are millions of people who undergo cardiac procedures each year. The teaching of postoperative rehabilitation protocols can be extensive and complex. Many of the patients are elderly and have some memory deficits. Others may have had memory compromised from the heart-lung bypass machines. Some of the topics that need to be addressed, such as when to resume sexual activity following a cardiac procedure, may be embarrassing or offensive to some patients. If presented on an impersonal Web site, the patient and family may obtain that information without embarrassment or offending their religious beliefs. If the information is not wanted, it can be ignored more easily on a Web site than if an individual is informed in person. The benefit of having the information available on a Web site is that the patient and family can access it multiple times, download it for printed copies, and if printed copies are misplaced, the information is still highly accessible. Web sites can gently lead people to highly individualized information by pointing them only to sites that fit their particular circumstances. For example, if a particular piece of information pertains only to male patients, the user can be told to go to a site specifically for males.

One of the potentially useful facilities that can be programmed into the Web includes reminder systems. Today, these are primarily exploited by annoying Internet advertisers. How many readers have some advertiser who sends them something every week or month? These are reminder systems and they could easily be applied to more socially useful applications. For example, how much does it cost clinics to phone every patient the day prior to his/her appointment so that excessive missed appointments do not bankrupt the clinic? Programs exist that could allow appointment reminder e-mails to be sent to every person listed on the clinic schedule for the next day or two. In fact, it would be possible (although possibly not desirable depending upon clinic needs) to make the entire clinic schedule an Internet application and patients could schedule their own appointments at any open appointment time. That way, a patient who wished to get in earlier could watch the schedule faithfully for a cancellation and obtain that earlier appointment. What might be very useful is to have the outpatient surgery schedule available on a password basis so patients could find their surgery appointments instead of calling the day before surgery at a particular time that may or may not be convenient for them. If that were possible, a list of pre-op instructions could automatically be shown along with the time of surgery and the time the patient should check in.

These are just a very few of the kinds of supports for patients that have been or could be offered easily through Internet sites. As nurses begin to collaborate in the design of Web sites for patient support, undoubtedly more ideas will occur to them that will both help patients and make the nurse's role in patient education easier. The Internet is rapidly becoming *the* source of information for Americans, and nurses can collaborate in designing sites that will ensure that patients have the right self-care information at hand when they need it.

Support for Orientation of New Nurses

During the past 30 years, the quality and depth of orientation programs have been greatly enhanced. In the 1970s, orientation might consist of a few lectures on hospital policy and a week or so of lightly supervised work. Today the standards have changed. Most hospitals have or are developing quite sophisticated orientation programs for newly graduated nurses. Such programs have even been extended to orientation of experienced nurses in a new hospital or clinical specialty. Traditionally, orientation was very specific to the hospital and even to the specialty unit within the hospital. Thus, each orientation program had to be unique. Today, most orientation programs are quite extensive. They include not only information about the specific unit and hospital, but also extensive competency assessment of clinical skill sets. Orientation must be customized to the nursing specialty, as well as to the unit and hospital. There are a variety of sites on the Internet designed to support orientation and clinical education. One popular site is Bob Bowman's site which highlights educational technologies (*http://www.user. shentel.net/rbowman/*).

For clinical educators interested in viewing a site that addresses online orientation, the University of Kansas (KU) site has an online clinical orientation page at: *http://169.147.169.238/comanual/*. This site addresses mandatory classes such as blood-borne pathogens, and fire and radiation safety. An online examination is provided at the conclusion of the content. A substantial amount of new-nurse orientation time is spent in classes on these types of issues, and a great deal of time and money can be saved by having new employees complete these courses online and then take an examination to verify competency.

Support for Nursing Continuing Education

One of the earliest aspects of nursing support to be developed on the Internet was CEU courses. Many companies in the business of providing CEU classes to nurses adopted the Internet as a medium for delivering their educational materials. Prior to the wide availability of the Internet, nurses' primary sources of CEU offerings were classes in their own hospitals, at local schools of nursing, at conferences, and from their professional specialty organizations. The courses at their own hospitals were usually provided at no cost and were convenient to the workplace. However, nurses often cannot get away from their patient care duties to attend classes. And when a nurse is sent to a class, another nurse must cover two patient assignments. This is not always safe for the patients, and nurses often miss classes they are interested in attending simply because they don't feel they can leave very ill patients for whom they are responsible that day.

The great advantage of online courses is that they are available around the clock, and if the nurse is too busy one day, he or she can always get online and take the course another day. Other advantages include: a) the cost savings in not needing a teacher in the room, b) the nurse can access the educational program in the comfort of his or her own home, if a home computer is available, c) if the Internet connection is available within the work unit, the nurse does not even have to leave the patient care unit to access the educational material, and d) people may learn better from courses available on the Internet than in traditional classroom settings (Lipman, Sade, Glotzbach, Lancaster, & Marshall, 2001). The disadvantages of online courses are: a) some nurses are not comfortable with this mode of delivery, b) the hospital may not pay for the nurse's class time unless the class is taken while the nurse is at work, and c) if the nurse tries to access the course from the patient care unit, interruptions can ruin the learning experience.

Nursing continuing education Web sites. Most nurses want very much to continue their knowledge and skill building after graduation.

In some states, they *must* obtain a certain number of CEU credits to maintain their license. There are an increasing number of companies that offer CEU credits through online courses, and these may be of interest to busy nurses who cannot easily take several days away from work to attend accredited conferences or who may have difficulty finding offerings of interest locally. A very small selection of online CEU sites will be presented here.

One site of interest is Web-CEU at: *http://www.webceu.com/*. This site has a wide variety of online CEU offerings ranging from 1–12 hours of CEU credit. There are classes on a wide variety of topics such as HIV/AIDS and breast cancer, and an EKG certification course. The NurseWeek site at: *http://www.nurseweek.com/* claims to have over 350 CEU credit course offerings. From that home site the user follows a series of hyperlinks to access their Web CEU offerings. An index of courses can be found at the following address: *http://216.155.28.162/nurse/ShoppingCart/index.cfm*. Another very useful site is Nurse CEU at: *http://www.nurseceu.com/*. This is listed as a sort of clearinghouse for online CEU course offerings. Hundreds of courses are catalogued at this site, and the topic categories range from AIDS to Wound Care, with many categories in between. Of great interest to many nurses is the compendium on educational offerings in the field of complementary therapies. There are reviews of therapies as well as courses on specific therapies. See chapter 16 for more information on continuing education.

DEVELOPING AND EXPANDING THE PROFESSIONAL NURSING NETWORK

One use of the Internet that has not been discussed sufficiently in the literature is its ability to allow nurses to greatly expand their professional network. Specifically, nurses can "meet" and communicate with a very large network of other nurses. Nurses have always identified colleagues who have special expertise in their hospitals and in their local areas. Communicating with these people has been as easy as walking down the hall, picking up the phone, or even meeting them at the local State Nurse Association or local Sigma Theta Tau chapter meeting. Many nurses have met professional colleagues at national meetings but keeping up those relationships has meant expensive phone calls or writing letters. The Internet makes establishing and maintaining long-distance relationships with nurse colleagues much easier.

E-Mail

Nurses often have met other nurses with nationally recognized expertise in a specialty at conferences. These relationships have been enormously valuable both personally and professionally. Yet, distance from
nurse mentors and friends can make maintenance of these collegial
relationships difficult. How many times have nurses thought, "I wish
my old Med-Surg teacher was here. She would know the answer to
this clinical question."? After attending a conference, how many times
has a nurse wished that one of the expert presenters was nearby to
advise the nurse on the best way to handle a problem? Today, keeping
in touch with other nurses is as simple as keeping their e-mail address.
Many of the author's students are quite surprised when they e-mail a
nationally known nursing expert and promptly receive a cordial, informative e-mail back. The students just cannot believe that the expert
has time for them. Yet, the experts are still nurses. They care a great
deal about other people—that is why they chose nursing in the first
place. Many nursing experts work in university settings, and often
universities have online directories through which the expert's phone
number or e-mail address can be located. Most nurses who have
expertise in a specialty are glad to hear from admirers and glad to
share the benefit of their knowledge. E-mail is a fairly quick and easy
way for most people to communicate about professional nursing
matters.

Chat Rooms

Another way nurses can communicate is through chat rooms. A chat
room is a capability that allows groups of people to send messages
to everybody in the group in real time. That is, instead of sending an
e-mail that one or more persons will receive later, a whole group of
people can have an online "conversation" at one time. Only people
signed on to the computer receive the messages. The chat room software transmits their messages back and forth. That is, the messages
are immediately (if not instantly) transferred to all people in the chat
room at the same time. E-mail is sent and waits in the in-box of the
recipient until the recipient retrieves the message. Messages are saved
on the server that owns the e-mail address until the recipient deletes
or erases the message. Of course, the recipient can save the message

on his or her own hard drive. With chat messages, the recipient must be signed on and in the chat room to receive the message. It is not saved anywhere on the Internet. Although the chat room participant may choose to save one or more or even all of the messages, typically chat messages disappear as soon as they scroll off the screen. Chat room software may offer the participant the option of saving a log of the entire conversation, and for online professional meetings, that is commonly done. However, casual chats between friends are usually not saved.

The advantage of a nursing chat room is that a large group of nurses interested in the same nursing issue can have a real-time discussion about an issue of interest to all. Uthman (1999) described chat rooms as one of the newer ways that the Internet is helping clinicians to expand their knowledge and communication with others within their discipline. The stimulation of ideas that can happen when one nurse reads the thoughts another has sent through the computer to all other nurses in the chat room can be a very powerful and emotionally rewarding professional experience. The disadvantages of the chat room are that the ideas are not preserved unless the members choose to print them, and that everyone must be signed on at the same time. Thus, timing can be a problem. People who are working during the time the chat room is meeting are excluded. Worldwide discussions are certainly possible on a chat room, but some members will probably have to sign on in the middle of their night. Despite these disadvantages, many nurses have enjoyed chat rooms, and have made wonderful professional contacts through this medium.

Discussion Boards/Listservs

More permanent versions of the online conversation are listservs and discussion boards. These two media provide software to support virtual conversations. The listserv is a special kind of software in which people enter items of discussion that are then immediately e-mailed to all members. In addition, members can sign in to the listserv software and view all old items. The discussion board does not e-mail items to everyone. It simply stores all messages so that people can sign on and read everyone else's items and enter their own items. Discussion boards are typically organized into different topics. Each topic is a forum and, therefore, the discussion board can support and organize several different conversations at once. For both listservs and discussion boards, people enter messages (called discussion items or, simply, "items") that other members of the listserv read. However, this technology was designed to retain all messages so members of the discussion could retrieve and respond at their own convenience. This format is wonderful for worldwide professional discussions. Different time zones are not an issue since everyone signs on at their own convenience. All items are retained for as long as the system administrator (owner of the listserv) decides to keep the message active. Chat rooms and listservs are typically accessed through an Internet-based Web site. Specific software is required to set up and maintain chat rooms and listservs.

Online Conferences

Additional Internet software and hardware now exists to support the types of online conferences that people previously had to travel to attend in person. Video cameras and microphones for the Personal Computers (PCs) needed in the conference rooms are inexpensive and extremely effective. Twenty to thirty people or more can join in the same conference. When a person is speaking, his/her face is filmed and the microphone transmits only that voice. Many executives who formerly thought that only face-to-face conferences could be effective have been surprised at the quality of video and sound available in today's PC technology. The few thousand dollars needed for investment can easily be recouped in a month or two from the airfare, lodging, and meal costs associated with travel.

This technology is now so cheap that it is easily within the budget of all but the most financially strapped hospitals. It could be used for clinical conferences with a nationally known expert clinical team when an outlying hospital encounters a rare disease. The audio and video technology is good enough to allow experts to both listen to bodily sounds and to visually assess patients at a great distance. Nurses in rural health services in western Kansas, for example, have used PCs with videocams and stethoscopes to listen to patients' chest sounds, to observe diabetic lesions, and to perform other assessments since at least 1995. This technology could be used to extend the hospital nurse's relationship with patients now that they are discharged so early. Although payment systems do not now support continued nursing assessment after discharge, that is a policy problem rather than a technological one. Such changes are more likely to happen if nurses show that they can prevent complications and expensive readmissions with less expensive, distance-based continuity of nursing care.

In all the online conversation media, people develop group courtesy norms, sometimes called "netiquette." In fact, a whole site devoted to teaching newcomers the proper etiquette for online conversations may be found at: *http://www.albion.com/netiquette/book/index.html*. Use of all these forms of media is becoming so widespread that there has even been a study of the group dynamics in these types of groups (Weinberg, 2001). As the 21ot century progresses, the Internet will become an ever more important communication medium for health care professionals— including communications among professionals, and between professionals and patients (Haux et al., 2001).

Identification of Experts

One of the most useful facets of the Internet is the ability to locate experts on topics of interest. When nurses want to find out who is an expert in a particular area of nursing, they have traditionally asked their colleagues who they have heard speak at national conferences, called a school of nursing to ask the faculty who the experts are, or looked at Medline to find out who is publishing in a particular field. But once the name has been identified, they still had to find the person. Today, both tasks can often be accomplished in one online session.

To identify experts in a particular topic area, one might first seek out authors of recent papers on the topic of interest by searching PubMed through the National Library of Medicine. PubMed typically identifies the author's primary affiliation (which is where the author is employed). Some hospitals and many universities now have online faculty directories where the expert's office number and address are published. In addition, an AltaVista search might well identify recent and future conferences in which the topic is addressed. Many conferences now put their schedule of speakers and topics online. The AltaVista search engine is likely to help the nurse find conferences. When the nurse searches the conference site, experts can be identified from the schedule or speaker list.

To locate an expert, a variety of resources are available on the Internet. First, as described above, if the expert is a member of a university faculty, an online faculty directory may provide the necessary information. Even without a faculty or staff directory online, if the facility has a Web presence, the facility's address and phone number are likely to be prominently displayed on its Web homepage. For example, if the nurse knows the expert is a faculty member at the University of Michigan in Ann Arbor, he or she may first want to search for the University of Michigan School of Nursing (SON) on AltaVista. (When the author performed that search, the first site was a directory of all schools of nursing in the U.S., which lists many schools of nursing by home state. Unfortunately, Michigan isn't listed. The second site listed was the University of Michigan School of Nursing homepage. On that page was a link to the faculty directory.)

If a faculty directory is not available, several other strategies can be tried. First, one can find the SON homepage. It is often helpful to erase all the specialty site portions of the address until one has the base address. Going to the university's homepage will usually help because most universities have links to their various programs and schools.

Ultimately, one may not find a faculty directory. It is then useful to go to an online phonebook such as QwestDex (*http://www.qwestdex. com/*). One can follow the directions to use the White Pages (residential listings) and identify the city and state in which the person lives. Qwest-Dex allows the user to include surrounding areas for a wider search in case the person lives in a suburb. One can also use the default business listings to find a phone number for a hospital or a university if the user could not find the facility's homepage on the Internet. If necessary, call the main number for the hospital or university and find the person through the main operator.

ADMINISTRATIVE SUPPORT AND QUALITY IMPROVEMENT NETWORKS

The Internet can be a wonderful source for organizational information. Some hospitals and universities have joined consortia that collect a wide variety of information on organizational performance. These data are stored in databases—usually relational databases that can be made available to members via a password. Most such databases can be searched if the user has some ability to formulate a SQL query. Although SQL is a query language that can be very complex and may require considerable programming skill, it is also a language that permits simple queries that anyone can learn through self study. There are a variety of books on formulating both simple and complex SQL queries available through from the Internet bookstore, Amazon.com.

One large consortium of university hospitals is the University Hospital Consortium located in Oak Brook, Illinois near Chicago (*http://www. radsci.ucla.edu:8000/frames/physician/uhc/index.html*). Other consortia consist of Catholic hospitals, Adventist hospitals, and hospitals located in the Appalachian Mountain area. These consortia can provide members a wealth of information on typical costs of supplies, case mix, death rates, numbers of incident reports, nosocomial infection rates, and similar information that can be used in administrative decision making. Members can use this information to evaluate their own cost and clinical performance, and to seek help from other consortium hospitals that exhibit a higher level of performance.

One area of special interest to multihospital groups has been performance improvement and quality management. While a hospital unit may use its own prior performance as the yardstick against which improvement is measured, a more demanding standard is using the best known performer in a formal or informal consortium of hospitals as the standard. Consortium hospitals typically have agreements that permit department managers to communicate and share ideas about how to best deliver quality care. When one hospital finds it has lower lengths of stay, infection rates, and mortality for patients with particular problems, other hospitals that do not have such excellent success rates can consult with the benchmark hospital. (A benchmark hospital is the hospital in the group with the highest performance indicator.)

Not all hospitals belong to a consortium. Even in those cases, the Internet can be a source of information about quality performance and clinical success rates. Some hospitals may choose to publicize selected quality data on the Internet. Medicare makes other types of data available. Conferencing and e-mail capabilities through the Internet make it just as easy for groups of quality management executives to communicate. Individual hospitals may choose to form "sister" hospital relationships, and the Internet makes distance irrelevant for these types of informal hospital consortium. Even without formal consortium agreements, the quality management departments of local, regional, or national "sister" hospitals can agree (with administrative approval, of course), to share information on quality performance and strategies and techniques to improve clinical quality in the various hospitals.

CONCLUSIONS

In this chapter, the benefits of having Internet access in the clinical care setting were discussed. The Internet can support nurses in both formal and informal information acquisition efforts. The chief advantage is the ability to use the Internet to quickly find information about medications, patient problems, treatment approaches, and other types of clinical information. The Internet also can provide nurses with a link to more formal educational resources such as proprietary CEU programs and mandatory programs such as the blood-borne pathogens annual class and exam. New-nurse orientation programs can be offered online either by the hospital itself, or by proprietary companies that develop such materials for sale.

The Internet can also be used to support professional nursing networks. Nurses can use these contacts to increase their knowledge of various issues in nursing, and to quickly consult experts on difficult clinical problems. Of course, nurse experts can more easily offer their knowledge and expertise to other nurses through this medium. The primary ways that nurses can use the Internet to support professional nursing networks are e-mail, chat rooms, listservs, and discussion boards. Various software tools on the Internet can even help nurses identify who is an expert in a particular area of nursing and, once identified, to locate and make contact with that expert.

Finally, the Internet can be used jointly by administrative and clinical nurses to improve the overall quality of nursing care, both in individual units and throughout the institution as a whole. Some hospitals have joined consortia of hospitals that work together to reduce costs and improve quality. Many of these consortia have begun making their information and supportive facilities available to members via the Internet. Even without formal consortium agreements, the quality management departments of local, regional, or national "sister" hospitals can agree to share information on quality performance and on strategies and techniques to improve clinical quality.

WEB SITE RECAP

Bob Bowman's Educational Technologies
http://www.user.shentel.net/rbowman/

National Library of Medicine
http://www.nlm.nih.gov

Netiquette
http://www.albion.com/netiquette/book/index.html

Nurse CEU
http://www.nurseceu.com/

NurseWeek
http://www.nurseweek.com/

QwestDex
http://www.qwestdex.com/

University Hospital Consortium
http://www.radsci.ucla.edu:8000/frames/physician/uhc/index.html

University of Kansas Clinical Orientation Page
http://169.147.169.238/comanual/

Web-CEU
http://www.webceu.com

World Sarcoidosis Society
http://www.worldsarcsociety.com/

Yahoo!'s Pharmaceutical Companies
http://cf.us.biz.yahoo.com/p/_health-majrrx.html

REFERENCES

Abidi, S., Han, C., & Abidi, S. (2001). Patient empowerment via a pushed delivery of personalised healthcare educational content over the Internet. *Medinfo, 10*(Pt 2), 1425–1429.

D'Alessandro, D., & Dosa, N. (2001). Empowering children and families with information technology. *Annals of Pediatric and Adolescent Medicine, 155*, 1131–1136.

Eysenbach, G., Yihune, G., Lampe, K., Cross, P., & Brickley, D. (1998). Like fire and ice: Consumer health information on the Internet and evidence-based medicine. *British Medical Journal, 317*, 1496–1500.

Fitzpatrick, J. J., & Montgomery, K. S. (Eds.). (2000). *Internet resources for nurses*. New York: Springer Publishing Co.

Fitzpatrick, J. J., Romano, C., & Chasek, R. (Eds.). (2001). *The nurses' guide to consumer health Web sites*. New York: Springer Publishing Co.

Goldberg, H., Morales, A., Gottlieb, L., Meador, L., & Safran, C. (2001). Reinventing patient-centered computing for the twenty-first century. *Medinfo, 10*(Pt 2), 1455–1458.

Haux, R., Knaup, P., Bauer, A., Herzog, W., Reinhardt, E., Uberla, K., van Eimeren, W., & Wahlster, W. (2001). Information processing in healthcare at the start of the third millennium: Potential and limitations. *Methods of Information in Medicine, 40*, 156–162.

Hejlesen, O., Plougmann, S., Ege, B., Larsen, O., Bek, T., & Cavan, D. (1993). Using the Internet in patient-centered diabetes care for communication, education, and decision support. *Medinfo, 10*(Pt 2), 1464–1468.

Lipman, A., Sade, R., Glotzbach, A., Lancaster, C., & Marshall M. (2001). The incremental value of Internet-based instruction as an adjunct to classroom instruction: A prospective randomized study. *Academic Medicine, 76*, 1060–1064.

Montgomery, K. S. (2001). Drug information and medication. In J. J. Fitzpatrick, C. Romano, & R. Chasek (Eds.), *The nurses' guide to consumer health Web sites*. New York: Springer Publishing Co.

Montgomery, K. S., & Uysal, A. (2000). Pharmaceutical resources. In J. J. Fitzpatrick & K. S. Montgomery (Eds.), *Internet resources for nurses*. New York: Springer Publishing Co.

Smart, J., & Burling, D. (2001). Radiology and the Internet: A systematic review of patient information resources. *Clinical Radiology, 56*, 867–870.

Uthman, E. (1999). To serve or listserv. Stresses from the field. *Clinical Laboratory Medicine, 19*, 433–451.

Weinberg, H. (2001). Group process and group phenomena on the Internet. *International Journal of Group Psychotherapy, 51*, 361–378.

Chapter 3

Skill Building and Practice

Mary Etta C. Mills

T he Internet and the World Wide Web offer a medium by which current information can be accessed for use in advanced practice as well as to build skills for practice application. Web-based programs and interactive software can facilitate the development of critical thinking and application skills through simulated client cases, virtual physical assessment and practice-based education and re-source referencing.

The Web is convenient and inexpensive, and has become an important tool for information acquisition. Over the past several years, the amount of health information available on the Internet has increased dramatically. Sacchetti, Zvara, and Plante (1999) suggested that searching the Web takes skill and knowledge, and Silberg, Lundberg, and Musacchio (1997) indicated that the Web may present a problem not because it offers too little information, but because it offers too much. The number of health Web sites is growing at a rapid pace. A recent survey showed that there are an estimated 3,000 to 4,000 health information Web sites (Voge, 1998). Some of these sites offer the opportunity for Web-based skill building and practice by nurses, while others are primarily directed to consumers seeking health information.

SEEKING PRACTICE AND SKILL BUILDING INFORMATION

Internet and Web-based information can be obtained using search engines such as Yahoo! (*http://www.yahoo.com*), AltaVista (*http://*

www.altavista.digital.com), and Google (*http://www.google.com*). These tools provide a means of finding specific directories and information. For example, "Provider Health" is a category within which there are 471 subcategories of nursing sites. Search engines can be helpful in locating information by identifying sites based on keywords, terms, or exact phrases that the user lists. If the word requested by the user is in the name of the Web site, the search engine will locate it. However, not every search engine will locate every site. If, for example, the user is searching for information on a specific disease or practice, the topic may be picked up by only one search engine because one engine may explore international Web resources while another may search more narrowly. A new search tool, 37.com (*http://www.37.com*) sends the search to 37 search engines and displays the results. Another search engine, Ask Jeeves (*http://www.ask.com*), permits the user to ask questions and provides assistance in identifying search criteria. Also, many search engines offer their own search tips, which are available as a hyperlink on their pages. Further information specific to using the Internet can be obtained through a Web site called Learn the Net (*http://www.learnthenet.com*).

Identification of information helpful to skill building and practice also may be obtained through newsgroups and Web discussions. Virtual communities have developed around the discussion of various issues in health, health care, and education. Some Web sites offer subscriptions to various mailing lists and participation in Web forums.

SKILL BUILDING

One of the most interesting and practical applications of the Internet is the capability of providing users with learning opportunities involving interactive exercises and virtual experience. The Web has become a tool for self-directed learning that allows expansion and enhancement of clinical skills. The advantage of this media is the ability to explore information of practical use and to gain experience where and when it is convenient to the user and as often as necessary until the skill is mastered.

An example of Web-based sites for skill building can be found by using the Google Web Directory and searching on "health > nursing > specialties." Some of the specialties included are community health, critical care, emergency, geriatrics, midwifery, neonatal, neuroscience, obstetrics, gynecology, pediatrics, and wound care. While these categories provide over 300 Web sites, only some of them supply actual practice and skill building opportunities. For those that do, presentations vary from narratives to interactive multimedia programs. Many are provided at no charge, whereas others involve a registration fee.

Sample Sites

There is a wide range of sites offering practice opportunities with great diversity of subject content. Only by conducting a specific search can the appropriate tools be identified. Some sample sites are identified in the following text.

University of Maryland School of Nursing (*http://nursing.umaryland.edu*) offers the RN–BSN program online, a 31-credit program for registered nurses. As part of the program of study, courses are offered in research, informatics, health assessment, community health, leadership and management, gerontology, and electives of the student's choice. This is a formal degree-granting program that enables students to gain skills and knowledge necessary for professional practice. Under the menu heading "Consumer Informatics" the University of Maryland provides free access to skill building programs that address issues such as emergency administration of epinephrine, respiratory assessment, emergency room triage, and virtual phlebotomy. These multimedia programs are interactive and permit users to practice decision making through case analysis.

University of Kansas Medical Center: Virtual Classroom (*http://www.kumc.edu/vc*) offers a virtual classroom as part of an online nurse practitioner program. Similar to other online programs, didactic instruction includes video and audio of patient care processes such as gait training, tutorials on blood gases, and self-testing.

Virtual Hospital: Patient Simulations (*http://www.vh.org/Providers/Simulations/PatientSimulations.html*), developed by authors at the University of Iowa Health Care (2001), offers case-based patient simulations for health care providers to practice skills. Simulations are offered in: Adult Critical Care; Adult Pulmonary Care; Carvedilol in Heart Failure Patients; Pediatric Imaging, Surgery and Pathology; Gastrointestinal Nuclear Medicine; Interpretation of Pulmonary Function Tests and Spirometry; Lung Tumors; Pediatric Airway Case Studies; Virtual Pediatric Patients; and Pulmonary Embolus Case Studies. The case studies include a patient scenario with interactive assessment and evaluation opportunities.

Central Nervous System Infection Cases (*http://edcenter.med. cornell.edu/Pathophysiology_Cases/CNS/CNS_TOCs.html*) were developed at Cornell Medical Center. Fourteen presentations are available with physical exam results, images, test results, clinical diagnosis, and outcome.

Eye Simulation Page (*http://cim.ucdavis.edu/eyes/eyesim.htm*) simulates eye motion (the eyes follow the pointer) and demonstrates the effects of disabling one or more of the 12 eye muscles and one or more of the six cranial nerves that control eye motion. This program was developed at the University of California–Davis campus.

Neurologic Examination (*http://www.medinfo.ufl.edu/year1/bcs/clist/ neuro.html*) takes the user through a complete examination with suggestions and acceptable shortcuts. This all-narrative program was created at the University of Florida.

The Dermatology Internet Service produced by DermIS (2001) (*http://www.dermis.net*) provides a searchable database for dermatological diagnoses and an image database and self-quiz.

Inner Body (*http://www.innerbody.com/htm/anim.html*) includes animations of various anatomical structures such as the mouth and throat, capillaries, cardiovascular system, ears, fields of vision, heart, lungs, nasal passages, and nerve and muscle connections.

Nurse Learn (*http://www.nurselearn.com/free_online_training.htm*) gives participants an opportunity to write performance objectives and provides self-study programs on topics such as competency validation, acute care, behavioral care, and long-term care. The offerings include availability of CD-ROM format, interactive self-study programs on topics such as blood-borne pathogens, environmental safety, and hazardous materials.

NURSENET (*http://www.graduateresearch.com/NurseNet*) provides Internet tutorials and a list of nursing discussion lists and Internet resources for nurses.

Concept Media (*http://www.conceptmedia.com*) is a fee-based program offering practice and skill building opportunities such as physical examination of the neonate, electrocardiogram analysis and intervention, and conscious sedation. Numerous educational videos and CD-ROM courseware are available in areas such as medical-surgical nursing, maternal-child, pharmacology, and gerontology.

Medsite (*http://www.medsite.com*) provides free interactive grand rounds on selected topics such as osteoporosis. A new case is presented each month. Other resources include fee-based CD-ROM software such as case files including interactive studies in language assessment, interactive pharmacology self-assessment, and an interactive case-study approach to nursing health assessment.

The Visible Human Project (*http://www.nlm.nih.gov/research/visible/visible_human.html*), developed through the National Library of Medicine's 1986 Long-Range Plan, is the creation of complete, anatomically detailed, three-dimensional representations of the normal male and female human bodies. The long-term goal of the Visible Human Project is to produce a system of knowledge structures that will transparently link visual knowledge forms to symbolic knowledge formats such as the names of body parts. Special applications are required for viewing images and are available on the Web site. However, a sampler of images and animations from the project are available online.

Nursing Interventions Classification (*http://www.nursing.uiowa.edu/nic*), developed at the University of Iowa (McCloskey & Bulechek, 2000), offers basic and complex specialty interventions with definition, label, and set of nursing activities that can be used in all settings and specialties. This Web site offers links with the North American Nursing Diagnosis Association (*http://www.nanda.org*).

Nursing Outcomes Classification (*http://www.nursing.uiowa.edu/noc/index.htm*) has implications for nursing administrative practice and care delivery in its provision of the first standardized language and measurement for nursing-sensitive patient outcomes. Using a standardized language facilitates the comparison of outcomes for large numbers of patients across groups, settings, or diagnoses. Sixteen 5-point Likert-type scales (*http://www.nursing.uiowa.edu/noc/overview.htm*) have been developed to measure patient status in relation to the outcome.

Web sites offering practice opportunities for nurse managers and administrators interested in learning more about budget and finance are more difficult to locate than are clinical practice sites. Government or educational settings produce most of these sites with a focus on reporting policy issues related to budget or to business programs or courses offering formal instruction both Web-based and on site. While not specific to health care, there are two Web sites that are especially interesting and may prove instructive of budget and finance concepts.

Virtual Economy Home Page (*http://www.bized.ac.uk/virtual/economy/*) is produced by the Biz/ed/Institute for Fiscal Studies and supported by a grant from the Nuffield Foundation. The model is based on the Chancellor's house and office in the United Kingdom. Sophisticated computer models similar to those the Chancellor and his advisers use to prepare the budget and to keep the economy on track are at the heart of this simulation. Case studies, economic policy, referencing, and a simulation model are available. The model allows the user to change fiscal variables and see the effect on the economy. While not specific to nursing, this simulation would be helpful to those trying to better understand fiscal issues related to economic policy development and could have some parallels to financial considerations underpinning health policy.

Simulations of nursing management and administrative scenarios outside of formal continuing education, certificate, and degree programs need to be developed by nursing professionals to facilitate skill building by nurse clinicians and nursing managers. At this time, most examples are driven by nonhealth care businesses and even these are few in number.

The sites discussed above are representative of the large and diverse number of available resources on the World Wide Web. Many of those listed under health and nursing headings involve skill building in physical assessment, critical thinking through case analysis and self-study, and testing relative to planning and intervention. They offer a means by which nurses in clinical practice can refine and expand skills related to the process of patient care. Administrators and managers may find it helpful to refer staff to the Web for additional refinement of knowledge and skills related to specific clinical areas.

STRENGTHS AND WEAKNESSES OF INTERNET-BASED SKILL BUILDING

The capacity of the Web to provide interactivity between Web-based practice opportunities and nurses has been growing. This resource offers increased access, as well as time and location flexibility. Most important, where simulations are offered, it is possible to learn and practice new knowledge and techniques in an environment offering the ability to repeat the skill as often as necessary and to do so confidentially. In that content can be offered using multiple methods of delivery such as text-based narrative, audio, visual, and interactive techniques, different learning styles can be satisfied. Similar content and experiences offered by a variety of Web sites can permit the user to gain different perspectives regarding specific practice skills.

Weaknesses of Web-based skill development may involve the potential lack of content depth and limited options for exploration of various application methods and expansion of skills beyond what is programmed. Content, by its nature of presentation, may also lack the necessary specificity for particular clinical environments and applications. In addition, the lack of interpersonal interaction in virtual environments may add a limiting factor to the application of techniques. Nevertheless, Web-based resources can be a valuable adjunct to the development and enhancement of practice skills and nurses seeking information may find this an effective means of expanding their repertoire of skills and network of professional contacts.

QUALITY

The use of the Internet and Web-based resources is still relatively new. While there are exciting developments in the field of virtual practice experiences through multimedia interactive programs, it remains important to evaluate the quality of the information available. Currently there are no regulations about health information on the Internet.

Articles published on measurement of the quality of information on the Web consistently cite three landmark articles by Silberg and colleagues (1997), Wyatt (1997), and Kim and colleagues (1999). Silberg and colleagues identified authorship, attribution, disclosure, and currency as relevant attributes to determine the credibility of information. Authorship is established when the authors and contributors, and their affiliations and credentials, are provided. When references and sources of content are listed, the attribution of the site is then known. Ownership, sponsorship, advertising, and underwriting need to be disclosed on the site. Dates of postings and updates need to be listed to determine currency. Wyatt (1997) added that the quality of the content must be assessed and Web sites evaluated for the reliability of structure, content, functions, and impact through inspection, testing, and field trials.

The Health on the Net Foundation (HON) is a Swiss nonprofit foundation that has created a Code of Conduct (HONcode) which they hope will raise the quality of information found on Web sites and identify those sites maintained by qualified people. The principles espoused by HON (*http://www.hon.ch/Conduct.html*) include:

- Provision of information by qualified professionals
- Support of information on the site by reference to source data and provision of a date of last modification

- Design of the site to provide clear information and contact addresses for visitors seeking further support
- Identification of commercial and noncommercial organizations contributing funding, services, or material for the site
- Identification of sources of funding from advertising and the distinction of promotional materials from original materials created by the institution operating the site.

Web sites displaying "HON" on their Web page have been judged to meet these criteria.

The importance of assessing the quality of the program being accessed cannot be over-emphasized. Misinformation can lead to serious errors. The capacity of the Internet for wide distribution of information makes accuracy critical. It is essential that users take the time to evaluate Web-based programs before depending on them for skill building.

The author of the site should be known in order to help determine and support the credibility of the site. Sites authored by professional health organizations such as the American Heart Association can be expected to provide accurate information. Likewise, health providers affiliated with large health care and academic institutions or nationally recognized health care organizations are likely to have high reliability. In any event, the name of the authors and their credentials and affiliations should be clearly disclosed on the home page of the Web site.

Information on the site should be current and a date of publication or revision specified. Because health information and health care practice is constantly changing as a result of new research, technology, and experience, Web sites should be periodically updated and a date placed on the Web site.

Web sites are developed for many different purposes. Some of these may include attracting business, generating revenue, providing a public service, or sharing personal experiences. The intention of the authors can have an impact on the presentation of the information. For example, use of particular medications and supplies for patient care as part of a Web-based case scenario may be the result of the company manufacturing and marketing them to generate increased sales. A site that is promoted by a company may also have a heavy focus on advertising. In another example, a site that shares personal experiences may contain information that is biased based on the individual's perceptions. The intent of a site may be somewhat determined by who is publishing the information. For example, Web addresses ending in ".edu" indicate an academic site, ".gov" indicates a government site and ".mil" is a military site. Frequently, but not always, ".com" is a commercial site and ".org" a nonprofit site.

There are Web sites that address the evaluation of Web-based health resources. Some information can be located at "Thinking Critically About World Wide Web Resources" (*http://www.library.ucla.edu/ libraries/college/help/critical/index.htm*) and "Quack Watch" (*http:// www.quackwatch.com/*). The latter site is focused on health fraud, quackery, and intelligent decision making.

Knowledgeable searching and thoughtful matching of needs and resources can provide a wealth of high-quality information and practice opportunities that promote the development of professional skills. Attention to the quality and depth of experience will be an important consideration in selecting Web-based programs.

SUMMARY

The Internet provides an expansive system of communication by which resource information can be located and accessed. Nursing professionals using solid search strategies can acquire accurate and quality information to enhance health care skills and knowledge. Many Web sites offer interactive programs simulating patient assessment, planning, intervention, and evaluation. The information, resources, methods, and skill practice provided through sites developed by professionals in academic settings, health care organizations, professional associations, and health related businesses can prove invaluable. Nevertheless, it is important for users to evaluate the quality of content offered and to consider the source of information including authorship, currency, accuracy, and purpose.

WEB SITE RECAP

AltaVista
http://www.altavista.digital.com

Ask Jeeves
http://www.ask.com

Central Nervous System Infection Cases
*http://edcenter.med.cornell.edu/Pathophysiology_Cases/CNS/
CNS_TOCs.html*

Concept Media
http://www.conceptmedia.com

Eye Simulation Page
http://cim.ucdavis.edu/eyes/eyesim.htm

Google
http://www.google.com

Health on the Net (HON) Foundation Code of Conduct
http://www.hon.ch/HONcode/Conduct.html

Inner Body
http://www.innerbody.com/htm/anim.html

Learn the Net
http://www.learnthenet.com

Medsite
http://www.medsite.com

Neurologic Examination
http://www.medinfo.ufl.edu/year1/bcs/clist/neuro.html

North American Nursing Diagnosis Association
http://www.nanda.org

Nurse Learn
http://www.nurselearn.com/free_online_training.htm

NURSENET
http://www.graduateresearch.com/NurseNet

Nursing Interventions Classification
http://www.nursing.uiowa.edu/nic

Nursing Outcomes Classification
http://www.nursing.uiowa.edu/noc/index.htm

Nursing Outcomes Overview
http://www.nursing.uiowa.edu/noc/overview.htm

Quack Watch
http://www.quackwatch.com/

The Dermatology Internet Service
http://www.dermis.net

The Visible Human Project
http://www.nlm.nih.gov/research/visible/visible_human.html

Thinking Critically About World Wide Web Resources
http://www.library.ucla.edu/libraries/college/help/critical/index.htm

37.com
http://www.37.com

University of Kansas Medical Center: Virtual Classroom
http://www.kumc.edu/vc

University of Maryland School of Nursing
http://nursing.umaryland.edu

Virtual Economy Home Page
http://www.bized.ac.uk/virtual/economy/

Virtual Hospital: Patient Simulations
http://www.vh.org/Providers/Simulations/PatientSimulations.html

Yahoo!
http://www.yahoo.com

REFERENCES

Kim, P., Eng, T. R., Deering, M. J., & Maxfield, A. (1999). Published criteria for evaluating health related Web sites: Review. *British Medical Journal, 318*, 647–649.

McCloskey, J. C., & Bulechek, G. M. (Eds.). (2000). *Nursing Intervention Classification (NIC)* (3rd ed.). St. Louis, MO: Mosby.

Sacchetti, P., Zvara, P., & Plante, M. (1999). The Internet and patient education-resources and their reliability: Focus on a select urologic topic. *Urology, 53*, 1117–1120.

Silberg, W. M., Lundberg, G. D., & Musacchio, R. A. (1997). Assessing, controlling, and assuring the quality of medical information on the Internet. *Journal of the American Medical Association, 277*, 1244–1245.

Voge, S. (1998). NOAH-New York online access to health: Library collaboration for bilingual consumer health information on the Internet. *Bulletin of the Medical Library Association, 86*, 326–333.

Wyatt, J. (1997). Commentary: Measuring quality and impact of the world wide web. *British Medical Journal, 314*, 1879–1880.

Chapter 4

Improving Performance of Clinical Operations

Trudy Johnson and Hussein A. Tahan

M anaging patient care safely and efficiently is an ongoing challenge in all health care settings. Health care and patient safety
reports during the past 5 years have emphasized the need to
reduce human error and improve clinical outcomes through the use of
decision support and various types of information technology (Bates,
2000; Kohn, Corrigan, & Donaldson, 1999). Focus on ensuring patient
safety and creating care processes and systems that reduce the potential for variance are highlighted by the 2001 Joint Commission on
Accreditation of Healthcare Organization (JCAHO) through its standards on patient safety and medical/healthcare error reduction. These
standards include requirements for appropriate communication of care
and the security of the patient specific information transmitted via technology (JCAHO, 2001). The use of technology enhances one's ability
to practice optimally, but also creates new challenges to ensuring
privacy and confidentiality, which are also regulated by law and accrediting organizations.

Despite the increasing demand for new technology, some organizations are slow to proceed with information technology solutions because
of the limitations in funding available to achieve the optimum work
environment. There is tremendous variability in the strategic planning
efforts health care organizations apply to implementing Internet technology (IT) solutions to improve efficiency and effectiveness of care
delivery. Many smaller community facilities may be able to automate

processes more readily if they can install a clinical information system without too much customization, but in a large and complex academic setting more customization may be required which can significantly increase the related cost. Additionally, the past several years have been fiscally challenging for many organizations because of the ramifications of managed care as well as the Balanced Budget Act. Variability exists based on existing computer infrastructures that make it more logical to interface multiple systems or attempt to upgrade older operating systems by creating a clinical data repository that is viewed via a Web-browser versus purchasing a newer release product. Often the organizations that have not relied heavily on IT for many years are at an advantage because they do not need to consider past investments when considering a current implementation. There are more options available now for clinical information systems, and the current systems are easier to use and meet more requirements for security than systems purchased five years ago. It would be useful for the reader to query the IT department in his or her organization to determine what strategic plan currently exists for information systems. With that information there can be a better understanding of the opportunity for innovation and improving practice through IT solutions.

Traditional clinical information systems such as laboratory results retrieval, admission/discharge/transfer (ADT) systems, and/or "coordinated" scheduling systems are now complemented by direct medical order entry, online patient record documentation (including assessment, interventions, and outcomes), point-of-care technology, patient tracking systems, and many other solutions. The increased use of electronic communication of orders, referrals, and diagnostic test results has enhanced the clinician's ability to ensure a safer, more efficient environment for practice. Applications that also enhance care processes include the use of an organization-based intranet, Web-based databases (internal/external), Internet-based sources of information or knowledge, and wireless technology. Each of these applications is discussed in this chapter.

REVIEW OF APPLICATIONS

Organization's Intranet

An organization's intranet (internal Internet) is a vital link to all employees throughout the organization. An intranet uses browser software to present documents in hypertext markup language (HTML) and graphic images that are accessible within the network of an organization, often without passwords. An intranet can also be designed to allow employees access via an Internet URL but may require a security code. Depending on the resources available to develop the intranet it can be a powerful tool for clinical, administrative, research, and educational purposes. Ideally, the intranet should be available at any employee's workstation in the organization. Furthermore, there should be kiosk-type workstations available in designated places for employees who may not have access to computers based on their category of work. For clinicians, all workstations in the patient care areas should have intranet and external Internet access.

Communication of vital information to employees can be done in standing Web pages, such as that of the Human Resource Department, or as special messages on the homepage (e.g., special communications such as a listing of medications for which there is a national shortage). Educational offerings and news releases are published on intranet sites; these can be augmented by electronic mail broadcast messages as well. Communication of new clinical protocols can be posted and can then provide links to important health care information that is published on the Internet to support evidence-based practice. Whenever new medication or clinical standards are published, the intranet makes a valuable communication vehicle, especially in a large multisite organization.

As a repository of information, the intranet should be the source for retaining hospital policy manuals that are available throughout the organization. This method of maintaining standards also ensures confidence that the document retrieved is the most current version of a standard (it is more difficult to disseminate hard copies to 200 people, for example, compared with posting the document to one Web site). The advantage of electronic documents is that you can hyperlink references and readily print pages that you want to carry with you. Some organizations are providing the same information that is available on intranets on handheld devices with smaller portions of reference databases or texts (e.g., the *Physician's Desk Reference*).

At New York-Presbyterian Hospital the Infonet (the NYPH intranet) includes Web-based access to two portals of patient-specific information. Both sites require log-ins and passwords to ensure security. One system that was developed internally is a data repository that allows the clinician to view data from multiple client/server applications from one point on a Web-browser. The data includes demographics, laboratory tests, radiology reports, notes and diagnostic studies. The second system is a vendor-acquired clinical information system that can be "viewed" from the intranet to read a patient's record with the appropriate log-in access. The benefit is to allow access to other users who are permitted to review the record (e.g., quality improvement professionals) but who do not need full access to the online system, thus maintaining the security and integrity of the system outside the clinical area.

Another application for intranets is the use of custom databases designed for use on a browser to allow multiple users to either enter or retrieve data. An example of data retrieval could include work lists or patient information that is fed from an interface to another system or from a download of a handheld device (e.g., personal digital assistant). This is useful when organizations do not have fully implemented clinical information systems that usually provide access to patient work reports. Thus, the intranet can be a useful tool to generate reports either from a data repository on a Web-browser or a customized database. An example at New York-Presbyterian Hospital is the use of the Discharge Delay database that allows for data entry on the patient care unit of information regarding why patient hospitalization is prolonged. This user-friendly format with drop-down menus provides for standardization of data and easy report generation versus a paper intensive method of collecting this information about patient care operations.

Advantages and Disadvantages of the Intranet

Departments can use an intranet to share with the organization highlights or achievements for the year, to recognize employees for accomplishments, or to provide selected hyperlinks to other parts of the health care organization's intranet or Internet sources a specific department considers important for its operations. The benefit of using an intranet is that it provides a Web-browser, user-friendly format that is easy to navigate and tools to work more efficiently. However, it must be acknowledged that not all staff are computer oriented and may prefer to read information on paper or listen to announcements. Electronic communication requires significant commitment to changing the organizational culture to one that accepts communication of information electronically. The organization must provide adequate access to computers to view information on intranets or in electronic mail, and must educate users who are not computer literate in order to achieve a significant culture shift. Furthermore, the IT department must maintain a system that is consistently available (minimal downtime) to give users the confidence that a computer can be as consistent and available as paper.

The Internet

The Internet has revolutionized communication technologies. Today all organizations rely on the Internet for locating, gathering, or sharing information, communication, and completing work procedures. The health care industry is no exception. Nurses, however, can rely on the Internet for providing better patient care in many different aspects, among which are obtaining information on certain diseases, treatment methods, or technologies, consumer education, consumer advocacy, and psychological or emotional support for patients and their families.

The Internet constitutes a major aspect of health care delivery whether directly or indirectly. Nurses and other providers rely on the Internet for information that enhances the delivery, management, and evaluation of health care services. Nurses and other health care providers may use the Internet mainly for evidence-based practice, expert knowledge sharing, performance improvement, adherence to the standards of regulatory agencies, patient and family education resources, and professional development. The Internet provides nurses an opportunity for worldwide communication and dissemination of information regardless of their geographical location or time zone, or the physical presence of an individual. In addition to knowledge acquisition from Internet sources, there are many databases available to query on the Internet.

Evidence-based practice. Evidence-based practice entails the use of the best available internal and external evidence to improve the quality of clinical judgments and to facilitate the provision of cost-effective health care. Nurses can engage in evidence-based practice by conducting efficient literature searches of certain topics, selecting the best of the relevant studies and research outcomes pertaining to the topic, and applying the results to patient care activities or in developing and revising the related nursing and clinical practice guidelines or standards. The Internet provides easy and timely access to databases such as MEDLINE, PubMed, PsychINFO, CINAHL, and the National Library of Congress. In addition, the Internet provides access to certain Web sites where evidence-based information is disseminated such as *http://www.guidelines.gov* and to journals that are published electronically such as the Online Journal of Issues in Nursing and the Journal of the American Medical Association. Moreover, nurses can access information advocated by professional societies such as the Critical Care Nurses Association, Sigma Theta Tau International, Inc. (STTI), and governmental agencies (e.g., CDC, FDA, Department of Health and Human Services).

Professional associations and agencies help nurses and other health care providers to ask the right questions, seek the right answers, and make more informed decisions. Some professional associations have developed their own evidence-based compilation of information such as STTI's Virginia Henderson International Nursing Library and the Online Journal of Knowledge Synthesis (available at *http://www.nursin gsociety.org*) that also includes a registry of nurse researchers and their areas of expertise and research. Governmental agencies also disseminate research outcomes and recommendations for evidence-based practice through publications such as those developed by the Agency for Healthcare Research Quality (AHRQ) (*http://www.ahrq.gov*) through rigorous analyses of the scientific literature. This site encourages the use and replication of the information. Sites such as the National Clearinghouse Guidelines (*http://www.guidelines.gov*) is an exemplary model of a search engine that provides specialty searches with a high yield of useful, current clinical guidelines for practice. Examples of AHRQ's publications are those in areas such as acute and chronic pain management, pressure ulcer and wound management, urinary tract infection in the elderly, and many others.

Expert knowledge sharing. Expert knowledge sharing takes place in different forums such as individual e-mail, group discussion via listervs or chat rooms, and personal or individual agency Web sites. Nurses can obtain expert knowledge by directing questions to authors and experts in a particular field of study or practice, and by answering questions presented by others seeking information. This knowledge can be used for defining best practice, changing practice and delivery of health care services, and developing standards of care or clinical practice guidelines. Expert knowledge sharing, similar to evidence-based practice, can be used to reduce variability in practice, control costs, and improve patient care and organizational outcomes. The knowledge shared is only valuable if health care providers integrate it into clinical decision making at the point of care and in a timely fashion.

Intranets can also be used to disseminate various types of information. Pediatric critical care units use dosage calculators that can be published on a browser. Radiology uses picture archiving communication systems (PACS) that transmit images on an intranet to be read either internally or externally. Common references such as the Micromedex or Physician Desk Reference online manuals for resources regarding medication administration can be purchased in intranet format to enhance quality and cost-effective patient care delivery.

Performance improvement and benchmarking. Health care organizations and nursing services are constantly engaged in improving organizational performance to optimize organizational effectiveness and success. They use performance improvement programs that assess, measure, and redesign processes to improve management of patient care services and outcomes. The ability to "benchmark" (i.e., compare one's performance to other organizations) is expected by current standards for outcomes measurement and performance improvement. The Internet plays an integral role in performance improvement especially for benchmarking of performance indicators for quality care. Many databases are available as a service to users who are members of an organization or consortium of organizations (e.g., group purchasing consortium), whereas other databases are available based on an annual licensing fee. Others exist solely for the vendor to make money. Professional associations and government funded sites also contain some databases that are accessible to the public. One must acknowledge that the data on sites in the public domain may have a longer lag time in publishing data than on profit sites. An organization can participate in providing clinical and financial data to any of these databases for benchmarking purposes. Such benchmarking databases are accessed electronically by participating organizations and allow the user to search for specific indicators of interest. Usually there is flexibility in the options for querying the database and report generation that will meet the custom needs of the end user.

The final notable use of databases and the Internet is the transmission of data. Examples include required data submissions such as pediatric immunizations to a city database over a secure line. Sending electronic files of patient data to state databases provides timely reporting of demographic data, including clinical diagnoses that are used for reimbursement and performance improvement. Participating in required performance improvement data collections, such as ORYX for JCAHO or the Homecare OASIS (Outcome and Assessment Information Set) data for Medicare, which are submitted electronically and receive reports in print, is another useful function of the Internet from a system perspective. Other organizations may receive data from the organization in print and then provide the reports via the Internet.

Standards of regulatory agencies. Nurses can learn about regulatory agencies and their related standards by accessing the latest information shared in their Web sites. Examples of these agencies are the Joint Commission on Accreditation of Healthcare Organizations (*http:// www.jcaho.org*) and the Commission on Accreditation of Rehabilitation Facilities (*http://www.carf.org*). Nurses and other health care providers can gain knowledge of regulatory agencies by e-mailing questions to representatives from these agencies, or by reading the latest information regarding changes in regulatory standards available on the agency's Web site. In addition, they can subscribe to the agencies' listervs so that they can receive information alerts in a timely fashion. Accessing and disseminating such important information is essential for improving organizational and nursing performance as well as enhancing adherence to the accreditation standards by ensuring the implementation of the latest changes, for example, the JCAHO's 2001 patient safety and error reduction or pain management standards. Other regulatory sites ensure clinicians are aware of important information about patient care and worker safety such as that provided by OSHA or the Centers for Disease Control (CDC).

Knowledge of regulatory requirements from HCFA are published online in the *Federal Register* regarding Medicare or HIPAA. Full-text regulations are available online, although many are tedious to read, and if the user is familiar with the subject, a summary usually can be found in a press release or public announcement. To make the review of JCAHO standards easier, the entire JCAHO manual can be placed on an institution's intranet site (license required). If someone has a question about a standard the reference page can be hyperlinked in an e-mail message and then read or printed by the individual asking the question or making a query.

Patient and family educational resources. The ongoing developments in electronic communication technologies provide a new venue for nurses in the area of patient and family education and support. Consumer-based information and health care resources available on the Internet are widely used by consumers and health care providers alike. Nurses can capitalize on this resource for better patient care delivery and to ensure adherence to the medical regimen. However, they are obligated to educate consumers on how to best use these resources. In addition, nurses can assist consumers in streamlining and simplifying such information because it can present an overwhelming task for patients and/or their families. Moreover, nurses can teach their patients how and where to access educational information and the difference between governmental and nongovernmental agencies and private, public, or commercial organizations, and the type of information they disseminate. It is recommended that materials be reviewed internally for literacy level and to find sites that also offer translations to Spanish and other languages. (Please see Fitzpatrick, Romano, and Chasek [2001] for additional information on consumer health Web sites).

Other resources available via the Internet are those that focus on patient counseling and emotional support. These resources provide patients an opportunity to communicate and network with other patients with similar medical conditions. Some of these resources are available either independently or as a part of professional and health care organizations. Examples are chat rooms, support groups, patient related home pages, or questions and answers using e-mail technology. The final area that is being developed is the availability of Internet access from the patient's hospital room via the television. Organizations are using bedside networking as a means to disseminate the internal hospital education network and also to allow patients access to the Internet while hospitalized.

Professional development of nurses. Continuing education resources for nurses are available online and are easily accessible. They provide a convenient and cost-effective approach to professional development of nurses that is not bound by time or geographical location. Most of the continuing education resources available today are accredited by professional societies such as the American Nurses Credentialing Center (ANCC). Continuing education resources include televideo and audio conferencing, and online case studies. Nurses use these resources to obtain educational credits required for renewal of specialty certifications. Today there are hundreds of professional societies and organizations that provide continuing education resources.

Nurses' use of continuing education resources is not limited to specialty certifications. Some seek out these resources for knowledge development and lifelong learning or to gain better understanding of the nuances of the profession and the discipline of nursing. Other added benefits of continuing education resources are maintaining competence and skills in a particular area of practice, and ensuring that knowledge of the standards of care and practice remains current.

Advantages and Disadvantages of the Internet for Clinical Operations

Some advantages of the Internet are:

1. Immediate accessibility of information compared with books and journals.
2. Eliminating the barriers of time and distance when attempting to access, gather, or disseminate information.
3. Ability to conduct a literature or computer search related to a particular topic that results in timely information from international resources and locations.
4. New information (e.g., documents) can be added to the Internet much more quickly than traditional publication media.
5. Messages can be sent almost immediately by one Internet user to another, or to a group of people regardless of geographical location, distance, or time of day.

Some disadvantages of the Internet are:

1. Connecting to the Internet is dependent on the availability of the server.
2. Documents available on the Internet are not always refereed/peer reviewed.
3. Information available on the Internet does not replace the need for traditional media and publications.
4. The Internet is not guaranteed as a safe medium and computer viruses may be transmitted intentionally or unintentionally.

Electronic Mail

The use of electronic mail, known as e-mail, is so widespread and popular today that every professional relies on it to conduct regular business functions. E-mail is the most common use of the Internet. It is the act of sending messages from one person to another using electronic media and telecommunication technologies. The transmission of such messages takes place via the Internet or a network. Electronic mail also is used to communicate between one individual and a group of people simultaneously, in which case it is called a listerv.

A listerv is also called a mailing list. It provides a forum for group discussion. Usually a mailing list is composed of a group of people with similar interests (e.g., nursing informatics) or professions (e.g., certified nurse midwives) who get together to share information through an electronic mail-based discussion group. Members of mailing lists can be from around the globe; however, they use the same language in their exchange of information. Mailing lists are asynchronous in nature and allow participants/subscribers to respond to posted messages at their own convenience.

Another type of mailing list is synchronous discussion groups (chat rooms) that provide an opportunity for real-time/concurrent conversations and discussions. Each chat room focuses on a specific topic or an area of interest. Chat rooms may be moderated or not. Moderators function as facilitators of the discussion and oversee the content and flow of information. They also possess the authority to disqualify subscribers who are disruptive or use obscene language from participating in a chat room discussion. Some chat rooms are oriented toward professionals such as nurses, physicians, or other health care providers; others are for consumers of health care (the patients and their families). Provider-based chat rooms focus on the discussion of topics related to the delivery of health care or the various professions. Consumer-based chat rooms, however, focus on topics related to health promotion, disease prevention, self-help, emotional support, and sharing of personal experiences.

Advantages and Disadvantages of Electronic Mail

Some advantages of e-mail and mailing lists/listervs are:

1. speed of transfer of information, that is, communication
2. ability to communicate the same message to a group of people at the same time
3. ability to put information and resources at nurses' fingertips

4. easy and universal access to patients and health care professionals
5. ability to transmit files electronically as e-mail attachments
6. ability to communicate with health care professionals at the patients' convenience without having to be present
7. providing patients with easy access to schedule follow-up appointments, or request information or advice regarding health care issues or treatments
8. dissemination of health promotion and prevention information such as newsletters or patient and family education materials
9. tendency to be informal in nature
10. participation in moderated discussions with book authors, experts, and authority figures in nursing and patient care.

Some disadvantages of e-mail are:

1. concern regarding security and confidentiality of e-mail messages
2. dependence on availability of a mail program and an Internet sever
3. the challenge to maintain compliance with HIPPA standards
4. presence of e-mail and Internet hackers
5. susceptibility of communicated information to abuse or mishandling
6. downloading attachments and files is dependent on comparable/compatible software applications
7. similar to postal mail, many e-mail messages are considered to be "junk."

ADVANCES IN TECHNOLOGY

While the Internet has had great influence on information sharing, processing, and management in health care, other (wireless) technologies have resulted in enhancing the industry in the area of patient care delivery and monitoring.

The Palm OS or comparable hand-held devices (personal digital assistants) are commonly being used by health care providers for keeping appointments, calendars, addresses, and telephone numbers. They also are used for accessing the internal or external Internet and e-mail. With special programming they can be used to interface with the scheduling system for patient appointments for diagnostic tests and procedures, to enter data in electronic medical records (documentation), or to collect data to be used for performance improvement purposes. However, use of wireless devices are not without problems. Access to the Internet from a wireless device and "beaming" of data can interfere with the radio frequencies of some telemetry systems.

Miniature testing equipment provides immediate and easy access to tests and results essential for identifying patient problems, diagnosing diseases, and providing efficient and effective health care services. The I-Stat machine, for example, allows nurses to perform point-of-care tests such as arterial blood gases, electrolyte measurements, and hemoglobin and hematocrit testing. Because of the use of the I-Stat machine, these tests are much less invasive in nature and are performed using a drop of blood rather than the larger sample required in conventional testing methods.

Another nontraditional monitoring method is the use of a hand-held device that is the size of a beeper to display cardiac rhythms from the telemetry system. This enables staff not to be tied to a central monitor. Other types of communication technologies used for better health care provision are wireless telephones and pagers that now allow for text messaging via the Internet. Special phones that do not interfere with hospital equipment can be used internally in a hospital "zone."

SUMMARY

Some questions to ask the organization are:

- What internal databases exist that can be queried for clinical or financial data about performance of clinical operations?
- What external databases does the organization participate in that provides comparison data to similar organizations?
- What is the hospital intranet used for and who controls what information?

The next generation of intranet and Internet development will continue to advance the accessibility of data in order to provide a more efficient and effective environment for care.

WEB SITE RECAP

Agency for Healthcare Research Quality
http://www.ahrq.gov

Joint Commission for Accreditation of Healthcare Organizations
http://www.jcaho.org

National Guideline Clearinghouse
http://www.guidelines.gov

Sigma Theta Tau International
http://www.nursingsociety.org

The Commission on Accreditation of Rehabilitation Facilities
http://www.carf.org

REFERENCES

Bates, D. (2000). Using information technology to reduce rates of medication errors in hospitals. *British Medical Journal, 320*, 788–791.

Fitzpatrick, J. J., Romano, C., & Chasek, R. (Eds.) (2001). *The nurses' guide to consumer health Web sites*. New York: Springer Publishing Co.

Joint Commission on Accreditation of Healthcare Organizations (2001). *Comprehensive accreditation manual for healthcare organizations*. Oakbrook Terrace, IL: Author.

Kohn, L., Corrigan, J., & Donaldson, M. (1999). *To err is human: Building a safer health system*. Washington, DC: Institute of Medicine, National Academy Press.

_____ Chapter 5

Staff Development

Julia W. Aucoin

_____

S taff development specialists have several roles to fulfill within organizations: educator, facilitator, change agent, researcher, consultant, and leader (American Nurses Association, 2000). The use of the Internet in staff development depends on which role the staff development specialist is fulfilling.

Most staff development specialists have gained their Internet skills at home, because hospitals originally limited access to the World Wide Web in order to keep employees from surfing the net when they should be caring for patients. At this point, staff development specialists without Internet access are demanding it so that they can fulfill all their roles, especially that of consultant. As health care organizations try to reach their employees, disseminate the latest federal guidelines, and utilize accessible resources, the Internet has become a vital resource for the staff development specialist to use daily.

APPLICATION MODELS

Orientation Anytime

The nursing shortage again has created a challenge for the staff development specialist. Nurse managers and recruiters have found it necessary to be flexible in terms of what future employees need (especially in terms of start date) and not rely on scheduled orientation dates.

Many nurses work in more than one facility and may not be available on the two Mondays a month planned for new employee's orientation. The computerized adaptive testing mode for the National Council Licensure Examination (NCLEX) allows new graduates to be tested when they are ready, making scheduling of hospital orientation a moving target. Additionally, as federal regulations and Joint Commission on Accreditation of Healthcare Organizations (JCAHO) guidelines continue to add valuable content to the orientation script, updating and scheduling orientation becomes more cumbersome.

Therefore, orientation, anytime, anyplace is one way to proceed. Creating agency-specific modules and placing them on a Web site makes sense when trying to reach an already working, part-time, weekends only, formerly employed, or busy new employee. In fact, it makes sense for all employees, except when socialization is an integral part of the orientation process. Use of the Internet for orientation can certainly provide the foundation and the required information for an employee to be successful in the agency.

JCAHO

Access to the latest JCAHO guidelines (*http://www.jcaho.org*) is important to the staff development specialist, as this person is often the internal consultant who helps departments interpret and implement the guidelines within their own work unit. Information about how accredited agencies have resolved situations, the latest sentinel events, and guidelines for accreditation are useful in this consultant role. Being able to clarify how guidelines are interpreted through use of frequently asked questions and direct e-mail can keep the staff development specialist from offering poor or expensive advice to resolve a problem. Many facilities purchase the accreditation manual and place it on the hospital network for access within the building and sometimes through the hospital Web site with password protection.

OSHA

The Occupational Safety and Health Administration (OSHA) is responsible for blood-borne pathogen training guidelines, HEPA mask-fit testing guidelines, and needle-stick prevention guidelines—all tasks that fall under the responsibility of the staff development specialist. Each summer, OSHA implements necessary revisions to these guidelines, and training plans must be revised. Access to the full report and interpretation through the Internet speeds up this process, eliminating the need for costly training and mailing of massive packets of information. Rumors and strict interpretations of OSHA's expectations are the norm. Therefore, access can allow for immediate clarification of information.

CDC

Isolation precautions change as more is learned about communicable diseases and blood-borne pathogens. The Centers for Disease Control and Prevention (CDC) is responsible for disseminating isolation techniques, guidelines regarding IV tubing and sites, and other infection control measures. The staff development specialist can be involved in policy and procedure development, but more often its implementation. Having access to accurate information about CDC recommendations can provide considerable cost savings in terms of preventing nosocomial infections and avoiding excessive expenses for overprotection.

Specialty Nursing Organization Resources

Training can be expensive, but so is developing new courses. Most hospitals develop a critical care course independently or in a consortium with other facilities to provide a constant supply of critical care nurses. The American Association of Critical-Care Nurses (AACN) has developed a critical care course that enables nurses anywhere to access the content and study standard materials. Each facility can plan a clinically precepted experience to facilitate application of this knowledge. The savings in terms of planning and teaching time far outweigh the purchase of the site license for the facility. Other specialty nursing organizations are working to develop such courses for common use so that experts can update this level of training centrally. These Internet-based courses can replace the more expensive (to manage) train-the-trainer options. This would be especially useful in topics such as fetal monitoring and chemotherapy certification.

Staff development specialists are often expected to provide quick solutions to both clinical and education problems. Networking with colleagues in the discussion forums provided by specialty nursing organizations is often a way to contact experts quickly and gain consensus on new practices.

Shopping for Resources

The staff development specialist must have access to the latest information, books, electronic media, and journal articles. For example, finding a good electrocardiogram (EKG) workbook could require a trip to the medical center bookstore or thumbing through several catalogs. However, by using a search engine to search among several book publishers or distributors, a wide array of available workbooks will appear. Often these include descriptions of the book and its contents, as well as pricing and ordering information. This is very helpful to the busy staff development specialist.

When shopping for videos, CD-ROMs, or computer assisted instructions, samples of the program are usually available through the vendor's Web site, so that a free demonstration can be accomplished without waiting or the need for special equipment. Since scheduling is not dependent on a salesperson's schedule, real-time comparisons can be made which aid good decision-making.

Finding journal articles can be difficult unless there is an in-house library. Yet with budget cuts, the librarian often functions as a consultant rather than a full-time employee. Managing the library can be a shared responsibility with the education department. The Cumulative Index of Nursing and Allied Health Literature (CINAHL) online database is available through subscription and to students at most universities. Abstracts and occasionally full-text articles can be available for downloading to disk or print copies. An abstract often contains the information that is needed. Several nursing publishers host Web sites that include access to recent journal articles that are available in a lengthy abstract or printed in full text for a small fee. As libraries become less of a physical location and more of an information broker, finding information this way will become the norm.

Products for Patient Care

Internet shopping has become quite popular for consumer use, but now as manufacturers see the benefits of providing an online catalog, health care equipment can now be viewed that way too. Again, the staff development specialist is often an internal consultant to the organization for problem solving and quality improvement. Being able to search for a product to improve patient safety or work flow without having to find a salesperson to send a sample or schedule a demonstration can be a valuable asset.

Evidence-Based Practice

Another role of the staff development specialist is to disseminate and utilize research findings. Specialty organizations offer a number of evidence-based practice products, such as continence guidelines with an accompanying teaching packet. Viewing public Web sites for posted information can also be quite useful, although evaluation of the Web site would be important so that any practices implemented would be valid and research-based. Sites available to the public include *http://www.guideline.gov/body_home.asp,* where information can be accessed through the Agency on Health Care Policy and Research (AHCPR) for a specific disease and *http://www.mederror.com,* a site that focuses on adverse drug reactions and prevention of drug errors.

Intranet Courseware

Computer-based software is often sold with a site license so that all the computers in a given facility will have access to the software. In order to make this accessible and cost effective, many agencies will distribute the software through their own intranet, an internal network open only to employees. While not the Internet, employees often see this as online education and will have a hard time telling the difference. This is a frequently used application of a network of computers for training purposes.

Hospital Developed Activities

One creative use of the Internet can be seen at *http://web.ucdmc. ucdavis.edu/edu/Resources/Resources.htm* where there is an interactive crash cart, demonstration of the use of a first-response bag, demonstration of restraint use, and access to an EKG rhythm strip interpretation exercise. Staff development specialists who saw a need to post information that is timely and vital for patient safety have developed these sites. With the aid of the hospital or health care agency's Webmaster, any poster-type material can be easily displayed to give learners a preview or a review of important content. In the case of the interactive crash cart, photographs of the cart were taken. By clicking on a drawer, the labeled contents were revealed. This is a great teaching tool that saves time and money—no need for a teaching cart and no chance of lost supplies from breaking the seal.

Additional creative ideas for implementation include using WebCT to place all testing for mandatory training online. Using the testing feature, tests can be automatically graded and feedback provided to learners in a timely manner. Also, lessons can be accessed anytime using video streaming, PowerPoint slides, graphics, and other colorful means of presenting content.

Army Distance Learning Project

The Army has recently embarked on a project to provide education in partnership with Price Waterhouse Coopers. The intent of the project is to make education available to all its members through distribution of free laptops and access to courses through 29 universities. This is another way of looking at the Internet as a staff development tool (personal communication, July 16, 2001).

Continuing Education for Nurses

It is often the responsibility of the staff development specialist to be able to refer staff nurses to reputable sites and useful activities in order to meet their individual learning needs, to prepare or maintain certification, or to maintain licensure. Chapter 16 (Aucoin) gives more detail regarding the use of the Internet for continuing education purposes.

STRENGTHS AND WEAKNESSES OF USING THE INTERNET IN STAFF DEVELOPMENT

As with any use of the Internet, it takes a critical consumer to know what is legitimate information and which Web sites lack credibility.

However, most of the resources that would appeal to the staff development specialist are sponsored by the government or professional organizations. The most common reasons for using the Internet in staff development activities would be to access timely and accurate information regarding health care issues. Weaknesses relate to the challenge of searching for information through a variety of search engines. Finding information is still a detective game. (For more information on quality Web sites please see Fitzpatrick and Montgomery [2000] and Fitzpatrick, Romano, and Chasek [2001]).

PRACTICAL CONSIDERATIONS AND NECESSARY RESOURCES

Medical graphics and digitized video can take some time to download using telephone modems. Most hospitals have Internet access through ISDN or DSL lines, which provide quicker downloads. Making computers available at a reasonable price as an employee benefit is a popular approach. Yet even more effective is facilitating staff nurses' use of hospital computers for education purposes. Setting up a computer lab or having a dedicated PC on the nursing unit would be beneficial in meeting educational goals. As more hospitals use PCs, policies on Internet access are being written to prevent abuse.

HISTORICAL DEVELOPMENT OF INTERNET USE IN STAFF DEVELOPMENT

The National Nurses in Staff Development Organization Informatics Committee has been actively educating staff development specialists for a few years. Besides monthly columns in the organization's newsletter, there have been two publications, *Guide to Getting on the Internet* (NNSDO, 1998) and a *Glossary of Internet Terms* (NNSDO, 1999). Additionally, educational activities have increased annually to include preconvention workshops and more concurrent sessions, such that each year almost 20% of the convention is devoted to electronic approaches to learning.

A couple of Web site companies, *http://www.healthstream.com* and *http://library.digiscript.com*, recently have been formed to assist hospital education departments in placing their work on the Internet, thus making it accessible to both their employees at home and to the nursing public for a revenue generating fee. As these companies become fiscally sound, more facilities will be inclined to enter into agreements with them. Additionally, there are companies that provide mandatory JCAHO and OSHA training via the Internet as well, for example *http:// www.net-learning.com*.

FUTURE DIRECTIONS

The learning curve is all that prevents staff development specialists from using the Internet in more creative applications such as that of the University of California—Davis. Partnering with instructional design specialists or graphic artists certainly will assist the staff development specialist in demonstrating innovative approaches to staff education. As the staff development specialist takes the time to learn about Web-based applications, more applications will become available.

Staff development specialists have an interest in working smarter, and use of the Internet for some of their planned activities would assist them in realizing this goal. As with many Web-based applications, the people responsible need to learn how to use them first in order to help their staff to use them later. At present, the Internet is a valuable resource of information to make patient care improvements, which is a vital role for the staff development specialist.

WEB SITE RECAP

Centers for Disease Control and Prevention
http://www.cdc.gov

Cumulative Index of Nursing and Allied Health Literature (CINAHL)
http://www.cinahl.com

Digiscript
http://library.digiscript.com

Healthstream E-Learning
http://www.healthstream.com

Interactive Crash Cart
http://web.ucdmc.ucdavis.edu/edu/Resources/Resources.htm

Joint Commission on Accreditation of Healthcare Organizations
http://www.jcaho.org

National Guideline Clearinghouse
http://www.guideline.gov/body_home.asp

Net Learning
http://www.net-learning.com

Occupational Safety and Health Administration
http://www.osha.gov

Resources for Reducing Medication Errors and Improving Quality in Hospitals
http://www.mederror.com

REFERENCES

American Nurses Association (2000). *Scope and standards of practice for nursing professional development*. Washington, DC: American Nurses.

Fitzpatrick, J. J., & Montgomery, K. S. (Eds.). (2000). *Internet resources for nurses*. New York: Springer Publishing Co.

Fitzpatrick, J. J., Romano, C., & Chasek, R. (Eds.). (2001). *The nurses' guide to consumer health Web sites*. New York: Springer Publishing Co.

National Nurses in Staff Development Organization (1999). *Glossary of Internet terms*. Pensacola, FL: Author.

National Nurses in Staff Development Organization (1998). *Guide to getting on the Internet*. Pensacola, FL: Author.

Chapter 6

Nursing Staff Recruitment

Maria L. Vezina and Michael Impollonia

Peple communicate through a variety of contextual mediums. The efficacy of technology such as the Internet with respect to communication cannot duplicate face-to-face interaction, but certainly can approximate this medium, especially when supported by two-way interaction and audio and video connections. On the other hand, information technology is advancing so rapidly that to ignore this advancement would be tantamount to isolation. Although the Internet is approximately 28 years old, towards the end of the last decade, it became a truly global network of information. The Internet is not only a computer technology but also a social technology. This revolutionary development has changed the world in only five years and, suddenly, we are all dealing with a "new reality" that has no precedent in human history.

What does all this have to do with nursing recruitment? In short, recruitment is all about communicating image, employment choices, service, scholarship, and learning about new situations and opportunities. Subsequently, new technologies such as the Internet, provide alternative approaches to the valued traditional methods of print media and advertising as well as person-to-person interactions and interviews. The development of the specialty of nursing recruitment should include advances in the electronic world promoting very public, virtual, and commercial vehicles of communication and publicity in order to remain competitive with nurses' and students' lives.

According to *delightinceptions.com,* a Web site and design company, some statistics about the Information Age include:

- Internet use equals video tape rentals
- 37 million people over 16 years of age use the Internet
- 25% of Internet users have incomes over $80,000 p.a.
- 50% of users are professionals
- 60% of users have at least a college degree
- average use is 5 hours 28 minutes online per week

When reviewing these statistics, it is quite clear that the registered nurse fits the profile. Thus, the importance of the Internet for the profession of nursing, in general, and nursing recruitment in particular, becomes critical as a communication vehicle.

INTERNET PRESENCE

For health care institutions as well as schools of nursing the development of a Web site and Internet advertising have become the "new" multimedia business card, brochure, and company presentation. A successful Web site design not only allows current and potential nurses to learn about your institution but, with the click of the mouse, they can learn as much as you wish to offer about your institution in real time. Initially, nurses can review historical perspectives of an institution, current profiles, important activities, and benchmark data. If you wish, nurses also may be able to search databases, respond to questionnaires, complete applications, order materials, and converse with staff members. With these activities in mind, the key components of a successful Web site include:

- Appearance
- Content
- Purpose

Appearance is what will attract nurses to learn about you and become engaged. *Content* will become your "selling" point—not only advertising what you have to offer, but also creating that competitive edge distinction and connection to "who you are." *Purpose* is the definition of your Web site—provided by distinguishing among the various professional interests of recruitment for career choices, memberships in organizations, applications for employment, acceptance into schools and educational programs, or finding opportunities for scholarship and research.

RECRUITMENT FOCUS

Nurses today want easy-to-reach sites that offer information about careers, networking opportunities, and methods to connect to prospective employers or schools. The advantages of online employment applications and the ability to send electronic résumés from home provide the advantage of "one-stop" shopping. The added opportunity of a "virtual open house or interview" is becoming an expected outcome for many interested applicants.

On the other hand, institutions want Web sites that are easy to understand, but which offer custom-designed features. Developing an Internet presence should be as easy as placing an advertisement without any technical jargon to wade through or hidden costs to investigate. Finally, institutions expect to realize savings since Internet advertising is less expensive than traditional print advertising and seemingly positioned more actively. Print advertising is restricted to the message conveyed at the time of the ad. Once portrayed in the newspaper, newsletter, professional journal, or convention materials, the intended publicity is unchanged and limited to the circulation of the medium. The Web offers the possibility of a dynamic flow of publicity, with unlimited change possibilities and an international exposure at no additional cost. Professionals and students alike look to the Internet as an online service for their job search needs. And with the critical vacancies that have surfaced throughout the country, nurses are marketing their skills competitively while hospitals are scrambling to come up with creative ways to recruit and retain staff using computer technology.

RECRUITMENT ACTIVITIES

The Internet has many functions of professional interest that relate to nursing recruitment: messaging with listservs; storage of typed words, pictures, sounds, animation, movies, and software programs; search and retrieval of stored materials; and procurement of materials both for educational programs and marketing of services.

Messaging includes electronic mail and mailing lists to members of news groups or special interest groups such as professional organizations and chat rooms. The rule that states "never post an e-mail that could not be printed on the front page of a newspaper" is golden for professional communications of any order.

Storage includes the ability of the uniform resource locator (URL) to be reached by Internet software so that users can search, retrieve, and download information about a prospective employer. Web sites add the context of multimedia to the competitive world of recruitment— offering unique experiences to interested candidates.

Marketing and procurement of materials allows nurses to hypothesize, critique, evaluate, and decide about joining any health care institution, agency, or school of nursing through the experience of a quick trip on the Web.

RECRUITMENT STRATEGIES

In planning for the recruitment and retention of staff in the 21st century, recruiters must recognize the upcoming dilemma of a labor shortage in the health care professions. In nursing, Alexaitis (2001) cites several contributing factors, among them the aging of the current nursing workforce and nursing school faculty, plus a decline in nursing education program enrollment. With a national turnover rate of 13.6%, according to a major survey by Phoenix-based Lawrenz Consulting, and with the Department of Health and Human Services predicting a national shortfall of up to 1.1 million registered nurses by 2020, nursing leaders must develop strategic plans for attracting and retaining competent nurses. These plans will include a journey into cyberspace in order to remain competitive with today's market. According to *medimorphus. com* (2000), 43% of nurses were interested in searching for a new job, mainly to secure better pay and improved working conditions and benefits. These remain today's primary motivators for seeking new employment. Employees are in demand, thus salary as a negotiating item is often the crucial deciding factor.

As for the allocation of recruitment dollars, according to a (2000) survey by *medimorphus.com* approximately 50% of recruitment budgets would remain the same for the coming year, although the need to find the right candidates for the right job would increase. As previously stated, most institutional budgets will emphasize salaries as the priority. Consequently, the more cost-effective method of advertising on the Internet has become *number one* in increased budget allocations for recruitment activities.

Other increased allocations, reported by medimorphus.com, are as follows:

Type	Percentage of increased allocation in 2001
Internet postings* *Internet includes company Web sites, job Web sites and other Web sites.	19
Job fairs	12
Recruiters/ headhunters	12
Targeting nurses	11
Print ads	10
General advertising	10

In general, however, recruitment budgets are reflected in a roster of activities listed by priority:

Priority	Activity by budget dollars spent	Percentage of budget dollars spent
1	Print ads/classifieds	64
2	Employee referrals	31
3	Internet use	26
4	Professional (trade) journals	22
5	Job fairs	22
6	Temporary employment	20
7	On-campus recruiting	13
8	Recruiters/headhunters	10
9	Open houses	8
10	Radio/TV ads	6

$n = 258$ Health care institutions

By comparison, the following lists the percentages of applicants' past and future usage of recruitment activities:

Recruitment activity	Percentage of past use by applicant	Percentage of future use by applicant
Print ads/classified	69	74
Employee referrals	45	54
Internet use	21	54
Professional (trade) journals	45	56
Job fairs	18	22
Temporary employment	12	12
On-campus recruiting	—	—
Recruiters/ headhunters	22	31
Open houses	6	17
Radio/TV ads	2	5

$n = 455$ applicant responses

Even though the greatest employment opportunities still seem to be in the category of print ads and classifieds among both employers and applicants, the potential of the Internet is where the future of recruitment is heading. *medimorphus.com* reports that in December 2000, only one in four health care employers recruited via the Internet, but six to ten health care professionals expect to use the Internet to find a new job. Clearly, the development of Internet recruitment strategies are in the future plans of all health care employers, since this is where the greatest opportunities exist given the modest or flat budget growth for this category in the future. In addition, according to a study by VHA Inc. (1999), online access has more than doubled in the past year among hospital employee groups included in the survey. Only 9% viewed online capabilities as unimportant. The researchers concluded that there is a logical correlation between increasing access and the growing use of online applications. Thus, health care institutions must be ready to produce online products and services to demonstrate quality and effectiveness, especially in the job market.

medimorphus.com identified the following types of recruitment sites and activities that are available for further development, sorted by percentage of usage:

Priority	Recruitment sites	Priority	Recruitment activities
1	Company sites	1	Search job databases
2	Job searches via Web site	2	Research employers
3	General job board	3	Research salary and benefits
4	Industry special sites	4	E-mail
5	Association Web sites	5	Network with professionals
		6	Apply for a job
		7	Post resume

WEB-SITE DESIGN

With the increased number of professionals navigating online, there is great pressure for health care institutions and schools of nursing to have a presence on the Web. According to Parkin (2000), the value of having an individual Web site is, as yet, unproven. It is best to have reasonable expectations beforehand and a thorough review of necessary technology and competent human resources to monitor these technological activities. Web site design, according to *delightinceptions.com,* includes many packages and features. Some components to consider include:

- Your own domain name (i.e., www.yourname.com) or a link to a domain name
- E-Mail Address
- Home Page
- Contact Page
- About the Company Page
- About the President/Vice President/Directors/Leaders of the Company
- Products/Services Page
- Web site artwork such as a color scheme, active graphics, logo incorporation, scanned/edited photographs, navigation buttons, bars and links

- Links to major search engines
- Account maintenance and customer support

When recruitment is the goal, creative applications attract candidates. Information about the institution and leadership as well as contact data are essential for successful communication and enhanced hiring outcomes. According to JWT Specialized Communications, an employment and marketing communications company, the second most visited page on a company Web site is the employment section. Thus, with any creative effort, there must always be attention to keeping information accurate and current, especially when recruitment is the focus.

CAREER SITES

For the promotion of career advancement and opportunities, it is important to consider that recruiting requires a multisite strategy because each site elicits a different audience. JWT Specialized Communications recommends that any Internet publicity plan incorporate a mix of sites listed below:

- The corporate site or company site is crucial to bring attention to your unique institution and employment opportunities. Conversely, your URL should be included in all of your marketing and recruitment vehicles to bring nurses to you.
- National sites have the highest traffic counts. Companies like *monster.com, careermosaic.com*, and *headhunter.net* are powerful communicators about jobs. However, the biggest complaint is that their e-mail is filled with resumes from all over the country and the world.
- Industry-specific sites are devoted to a particular practice area like nursing (*www.springnet.com*), or a specialty area within nursing such as critical care (*www.aacn.org*), or the operating room (*www.aorn.org*). These sites drive very focused traffic and are highly recommended.
- Regional sites are career sites that serve cities, states, and regions. These sites are ideal for attracting local candidates and they have less traffic than national sites. Regional sites are a very targeted way of collecting resumes for consideration. Examples

include *www.nursingspectrum.com, www.nurseweek.com,* and *nursinghands.com.*

- College sites are hosted by college and university career centers. New graduates and alumnae are the focus for access to the listed career opportunities.

With all the sites described above, JWT Specialized Communications recommends the use of banner ads and corporate profiles with direct links to the corporate or company site rather than individual job postings. At this time, they also recommend that 20–25% of the recruitment budget be targeted to the Internet, again keeping in mind a multisite application for the greatest exposure and success.

EVALUATION OF CAREER SITES

According to a study by the Internet Business Network (2001), there are 10 easy questions you can use to evaluate a site, including:

- What do you think of the site? Is it professional in appearance, easy to navigate, and appropriate to the intended message?
- Are there relevant jobs and content on the site? Are the job postings limited only to entry-level positions, or is there a broad base of career opportunities? Job seekers will tend to visit the site with the most diverse selection.
- Who else is in on the site? Knowing the competition is an important consideration for choosing a site for advertisement. The presence of other companies may dissuade or persuade you from joining the same site.
- How difficult is the career site to find? Determine how many visits the site receives each month so as to determine the traffic and decide whether it is worth joining.
- What are candidates looking for on the site? Gather some initial data about the kind of jobs that were most targeted at the site. This will help you decide whether or not to join in.
- How flexible is the pricing? Ask about trial periods, banner or resume database promotions, or length of contracts. Setting up relationships with the online media representatives is crucial.
- What are the site's marketing efforts? Does the site have their own marketing campaign and are they focused on career opportunities and employer profiles?

- What is the size of the resume database? The quality of the resume database on a job site is also important to investigate. How old the resumes are, the size of the pool, and how easy the database is to search, are important considerations.
- Is the site ready for the future? There are always improved technological features to be aware of. Before signing a contract, make sure that investment in a program will not result in later losses for a vehicle that is no longer popular or effective.
- How good is the site's functionality? Determine how many clicks it takes to locate a job or research an employer profile. Is the site designed so that visitors will come back for more, or are the download and search processes so cumbersome and time-consuming, that a visitor will never return?

THE NEW-AGE RESUME

The purpose of a resume is to provide a clear synopsis of your educational and professional accomplishments. But today, the format you choose, including electronic, may well be as crucial as any of your qualifications in getting the job you desire. According to Farella (2001), a growing number of employers are now using automated applicant tracking systems—databases that electronically store, compare, and retrieve the resumes of prospective employees. This system works very much like the automated systems used to do literature searches. The tracking system retrieves those resumes entered into a database that contain the keywords specified. Thus, to be considered for many types of positions, it is up to the job seekers to get their resumes into the major databases used by health care institutions. The basic data in an online resume is the same as in a traditional one, but you may need to become familiar with the key words employers use in their searches. You can obtain cues about key words by scanning online job listing sites. Technical ground rules for creating online resumes are another major consideration. The content of your resume will not matter much if a recruiter is unable to download it. According to Farella (2001), it becomes necessary to follow a few ground rules:

- Choose a common, readable typeface such as Arial or Times New Roman.
- Use at least 12- or 14-point type.

- Use boldface and capital letters for emphasis rather than graphics, shading, italics, or underlining.
- When e-mailing your resume to a Web site, follow the requirements of that database such as specified margins or using spaces instead of tabs.
- Convert your document to text only or to a rich text format (RTF) which can be read by all computers.
- Read user guidelines thoroughly before posting your resume online.
- Protect your privacy by citing previous or current employers in general terms.
- Keep track of your databases so that you do not have multiple resumes in a single database.

Many employers are starting to locate candidates through automated applicant tracking systems. While the traditional paper resume is not in danger of becoming obsolete any time soon, marketing yourself with an electronic resume becomes an added dimension of any job search. This technology can only increase your chances of interviewing for, and subsequently receiving, the ultimate job offer.

SUMMARY

Information technology is becoming a very rich and efficient infrastructure for nursing recruitment operations. The information transfer process of the 21st century is extremely powerful and having the right technology at the right time strongly influences recruiting competent, qualified people. Use of the Internet to the fullest may well become the competitive edge for many health care institutions, providing avenues for advertisement, promoting external and internal communication with nurses, and establishing new standards for recruitment and retention of staff.

WEB SITE RECAP

American Association of Critical Care Nurses
http://www.aacn.org

Association of Perioperative Registered Nurses
http://www.aorn.org

Careermosaic.com
http://www.careermosaic.com

Delightinceptions.com
http://www.delightinceptions.com

Headhunter.net
http://www.headhunter.net

Internet Business Network
http://www.interbiznet.com

Medimorphus.com
http://www.medimorphus.com

Monster Jobs
http://www.monster.com

Nurseweek
http://www.nurseweek.com

Nursing Spectrum
http://www.nursingspectrum.com

Nursinghands.com
http://www.nursinghands.com

Springnet
http://www.springnet.com

REFERENCES

Alexaitis, I. (2001). Planning for Recruitment and Retention. *Nursing Spectrum.* [Online]. Available: *www.nursingspectrum.com.*
delightinceptions.com (2001). Web Site Design and Hosting. [Online]. Available: *www.delightinceptions.com.*
Farella, C. (2001). Interviewing for success. *Imprint*, 40–41.
Internet Business Network (2001). Electronic Recruiting Index. [Online]. Available: *www.interbiznet.com.*
JWT Specialized Communications (2001). Media Recommendation/Rationale. [Online]. Available: *www.jwtworks.com.*

medimorphus.com (2000). The Healthcare Profession Job Market: What Positions Are Employers Seeking to Fill? Which Professionals Are Looking for New Jobs? [Online]. Available: *www.medimorphus.com.*

Parkin, S. L. (2000). Web site marketing: What's your choice? *Nursing Homes, 49*(11), 35.

VHA, Inc. (1999). Hospital Staffs Increase Internet Use. [Online]. Available: *www.vha.com.*

Chapter **7**

Home Care Considerations

Georgia Narsavage

H ome care provides the opportunity to observe the patient in his or her daily environment. Traditional patient observation has been enhanced through communication with health care specialists. Health care specialists no longer are limited to areas needing direct access. Telecommunications and the World Wide Web have been used progressively to expand the role of specialists in home care for the past decade. Sweeney and Skiba (1995) defined telecommunications as wire, optical devices, radio, or other electromagnetic methods to send and receive voice, video, or data information. Home care nurses have frequently used the simplest telecommunication system— the telephone—to communicate over wide distances. Today, RNs and APNs are increasingly using computer capabilities to expand the variety and type of information that can be accessed and shared, and sending digital images provides further opportunities for expert assessment based on the idea that one picture can communicate more than many words.

The Internet has opened opportunities for access to written information, reference materials, expert opinion, and individual education in both urban and remote areas of the world. In the home setting, electronic mail (e-mail) facilitates communication between health care professionals and their patients. E-mail enhances communication between professionals themselves and between professional organizations and nurses. Interactive problem solving is facilitated through the listserv of organizations by allowing difficult cases to be posted for consultation—

often without charge. Further development has the potential to provide site-of-care options that bring the expert to the bedside without moving the bed from the patient's home. Intelligent monitoring systems can reflect the patient's health status and alert distant health care professionals to the need for follow-up. Cost analysis and research in the use of the Internet in home care is the logical next step.

CURRENT MODELS OF PRACTICE IN HOME CARE

There are multiple applications of the Internet in the home care practice setting. Communication with others includes e-mail/Internet discussion between nurses/APNs and other care providers, as well as problem solving of clinical cases on bulletin boards locally, nationally, and internationally. The Internet is being used to obtain coping support from others dealing with similar problems, and for teleconsultation, teleconferencing, telereporting, record storage, and telemonitoring.

Access to reference resources is an important support mechanism for home care. Staff members in the field are able to connect to the home care office to retrieve patient information, to be informed of administrative decisions, to research data, and to obtain current articles. Home care agency personnel in and out of the office can perform searches of the literature from libraries at universities, state-wide links, the National Library of Medicine, and internationally.

STRENGTHS AND WEAKNESSES OF USING THE INTERNET IN HOME CARE NURSING

The benefits of using the Internet in home care nursing include the efficacy of using home-recorded data for current information access and using intelligent systems so that home care RNs and APNs can suggest solutions based on current recommended treatment guidelines. By using the Internet for assessment and interventions, patient updates such as for those with diabetes, heart failure, asthma, and chronic obstructive pulmonary disease (COPD) can be readily accessed from the home. Access to this information can reduce anxiety for patients and caregivers, and improve access to specialists who can assess and intervene, provide education, and set visit dates from a distance.

Caregivers can receive ongoing support 24 hours a day with Internet access. Data can be collected and analyzed in a timely way for both process and outcome data. It is possible to produce current reports for insurers, employers, and the public from such databases. Additionally, others have found this type of information system can assist in meeting Joint Commission Standards for Information Management (Bradley, 1995).

It is not easy to introduce an Internet system into traditional care settings such as the home. Weaknesses of such systems include cost and time for learning that can be an uphill curve if staff are not familiar with computers. Additionally, video transmissions from the home can be unclear due to lighting, presentation angles, and lack of skills of the patient and family at home. Phone connections may also present technical difficulties. The potential for information overload can reduce productivity. Finally, there is a need to control access for security of data and secure password systems require frequent updating—possibly adding frustration for the users.

PRACTICAL CONSIDERATIONS AND NECESSARY RESOURCES

Attention to practical details and obtaining adequate resources can facilitate successful system implementation. Upfront planning and intersystem compatibility are essential because once a system is purchased, upgrading the system is difficult, if not prohibitively expensive. Monitoring devices (scales, blood pressure monitors, etc.) can transmit data regularly, but need adaptive devices that may be costly initially. Patients and families have transmitted weight and vital signs by telephone, but teaching them how to use the equipment can be time consuming. Nurses at the office can monitor the transmitted data and compare their findings with physician or APN established parameters, and phone patients if variances exist; however, knowledge of how to support patient responses can be a problem if guidelines do not specifically address the follow-up care that is needed.

Rowland and Rowland (1997) identified three components that must be present for the home computer system to work: "a longitudinal computerized patient record," a "common nursing language" for records (OASIS is fast becoming the standard system for home care), and "widespread information networks" (pp. 308–309).

HISTORICAL DEVELOPMENT OF INTERNET USE IN HOME CARE

Artificial intelligence capabilities involving computerized care have been proposed as an optimal system for decision support since the 1980s (Brennan, 1988). Programmed protocols for complex decision-making has provided a practical and cost-effective method of implementing practice guidelines (McDonald et al., 1984) and a paperless home monitoring program has been demonstrated as feasible (Finkelstein et al., 1993). Nurses' use of point-of-service (POS) computers has been increasingly noted over the past decade. In a quality improvement study designed to improve clinical documentation, Quigley, Mathis, and Nodhturft (1994) used a POS computerized documentation system to individualize care. Documentation analysis provided "cues" for the bedside nurse, developing 93% compliance on admission and reassessment based on the Joint Commission on Accreditation of Healthcare Organizations Standards for Nursing Care (1992). They proposed that the next step should be to program the computer to use Standards of Practice as a basis for adjusting care planning. Nurses perceived the technical feasibility and practicality of staff nurses using computers for POS care positively.

A recent report by Allen and Englebright (2000) described improvement of a computerized nursing documentation system in an inner city area by using the intelligent analysis capabilities of the computer to streamline data analysis for planning care and POS decision-making. Standards of Practice with nonredundant data collection screens and 12 to 14 associated interventions were built into systems for each clinical area such as the Medical/Surgical Care Area within the hospital. Age-related needs were integrated and used in terms of "suggested" computer care guidelines. In addition to the time saved by the parsimonious data collection, multidisciplinary use of bedside computers was considered a critical aspect of an effective and efficient information system. Data were downloaded to an internal network that was used to monitor compliance with quality standards and track improvements in the process of care. Nurses and managers unanimously wished to continue using the POS system. This type of intelligent analysis system has been adapted to the home care agency through home and back communication.

Information technology developments for home care are also being developed internationally. In Finland, Korhonen and colleagues (2001) described TERVA, their wellness monitoring system for home use. TERVA works on a laptop computer to provide measures of vital signs and other variables that reflect the individual's health status, confirmed by the patient's self-recorded diary that is also maintained on the computer. This system has been proposed as a way to discharge patients without the extensive need for direct home care. One concern is that the age of many patients with chronic illness may discourage them from using the equipment.

Tan (1995) described three benefits of a computerized system. These included the ability to: (a) enhance operational efficiency, (b) promote innovation, and (c) provide timely resources based on relevant and current data. These apply to the home setting as RNs and APNs use both on-site and distant computer networks/systems to communicate, obtain information, and obtain decisional support.

COST ANALYSIS

As home care providers assess patterns of care that result in obtaining positive outcomes and are cost-effective while also maintaining quality care and client/family satisfaction, the use of computer intelligence has increased. Home care today is generally paid under a prospective payment system (PPS) in a capitated amount based on the patient's home health related grouping (HHRG); knowing the effect of particular combinations of interventions and at what time they can be most effective can promote fiscally responsible decision making when resources are limited. When data are collected over time, a home care agency has the opportunity to identify what treatments are effective in varied situations for different patients with different diseases and levels of severity. Quality control can be automated to support obtaining valid data, because the computer system can prompt the RN to reevaluate the data if it is outside the set of expected parameters.

Home care agencies that have remained competitive since the implementation of PPS have collected the mandated outcome and assessment information set (OASIS) data via an automated point-of-care system for home care nurses (Medicare and Medicaid Programs, 1999). The use of the Internet to "download" the data directly from the patients' homes and then access the data through secure systems can increase accessibility and decrease nurses' time. It has become possible for agencies to develop guidelines and recommendations for implementation measures in patient groups—a valuable tool to both new practitioners and RNs with little previous opportunity to develop expertise in specialty patient care areas. Benchmarks that have been identified for intermediate and final expected points of care can guide the home care nurse and provide payers with information on outcomes obtained. APNs can provide expert consultations with nurses at the bedside through carefully planned guidelines based on previous evidence of effectiveness. Using intranet systems to promote privacy and confidentiality, and adding "relational databases" that include information on similar patient situations, can enhance outcome analysis and facilitate identifying care patterns that are effective. Litzelman, Dittus, Miller, and Tierney (1993) found that having physicians respond to computerized reminders improved their compliance with preventive care protocols. This reminder system has implications for both APN and RN nurse assessment and care planning and charting, and has in fact been built into the OASIS data systems in home care. As patient homes are increasingly wired for home Internet access, patients can perform self-monitoring activities, report results (such as peak-flow measures for people with asthma), and complete functional status or symptom surveys.

RESEARCH SUPPORT FOR INTERNET USE IN HOME CARE SETTINGS

Noone, Cavanaugh, and McKillip (1995) reported on the feasibility and practicality of using a computerized POS system for home health care. All clinical standards were met based on the 1991 Community Health Accreditation Program Standards of Excellence (2001) after agency home care staff nurses implemented a computerized charting system. Computers were used to automate collection of assessment and evaluation data, and to promote consistent documentation. Nurses who used the system reported that they would not want to return to manual charting. Affordability was reported using lightweight computers that were less expensive than laptops. Chart data were downloaded at the end of each day by returning to the agency. Automated quality control mechanisms were used to assure the validity of the data. They suggested that markers of intermediary and final outcomes of care could provide benchmarks to providers and payers. Future developments may simulate research on benefits of computerized nursing support that personalizes in-home access to information and capitalizes on the availability of Internet resources (Brennan, Caldwell, Moore, Sreenath, & Jones, 1998).

Finkelstein's work, as reported in *Heart and Lung* (1993), and that of his colleagues (Lindgren et al., 1997) has demonstrated the efficacy of using home-recorded data in a paperless electronic monitoring system to improve the continuity of in-home care. Additionally, in his current study (2RO1NR02128-04A1), the early detection of lung transplant rejection/infection is supported by a computerized decision system based on previously researched algorithms. Patients send the data through a modem connection directly to the laboratory, analysis of the data is performed, and data that are outside set parameters trigger a notification system independently.

FUTURE DIRECTIONS

Intervention research with a cost-benefit analysis to determine the effects of home monitoring by specialists at a distance compared with in-home care interventions or self-care focus for distance monitoring could answer questions related to how intelligently the systems are used.

Few options for intelligent decision-support systems for nursing have been developed to date; this is the logical next step for intelligent assessment data collection systems. Collaborative practice demands care delivery that can adapt, often quickly, to accommodate changes in the patient's condition. Computers can facilitate this change.

REFERENCES

Allen, J., & Englebright, J. (2000). Patient-centered documentation: An effective and efficient use of clinical information systems. *Journal of Nursing Administration, 30*(2), 90–95.

Bradley, J. (1995). Management of information: Analysis of the Joint Commission's Standards for Information Management. *Topics in Health Information Management, 16*(2), Preamble.

Brennan, P. (1988). DSS, ES, AI: The lexicon of decision support. *Nursing and Health Care, 9,* 501–503.

Brennan, P. F., Caldwell, B., Moore, S. M., Sreenath, N., & Jones, J. (1998). Designing heart care: Custom computerized home care for patients recovering from CABG surgery. *American Medical Informatics Association Journal,* 381–385.

CHAP: Community Health Accreditation Program (2001). The Standards of Excellence. Available at *http://www.chapinc.org/chap-soe.html*

Finkelstein, S., Lindgren, B., Prasad, B., Snyder, M., Edin, C., Wielinski, C., & Hertz, M. (1993). Reliability and validity of spirometry measurements in a paperless home monitoring diary program for lung transplantation. *Heart & Lung, 22,* 523–533.

JCAHO Standards for Nursing Care (1992). *Hospital accreditation standards.* Chicago: Author.

Korhonen, I., Iavainen, T., Lappalainen, R., Tuomisto, T., Koobi, T., Pentikainen, V., Tuomisto, M., & Turjanmaa, V. (2001). TERVA: System for long-term monitoring of wellness at home. *Telemed Journal of E Health, 7,* 61–72.

Lindgren, B. R., Finkelstein, S. M., Prasad, B., Dutta, P., Killoren, T., Scherber, J., Stibbe, C. L. E., Snyder, M., & Hertz, M. I. (1997). Determination of reliability and validity in home monitoring data of pulmonary function tests following lung transplantation. *Research in Nursing & Health, 20,* 539–550.

Litzelman, D. K., Dittus, R. S., Miller, M. E., & Tierney, W. M. (1993). Requiring physicians to respond to computerized reminders improves their compliance with preventive care protocols. *Journal of General Internal Medicine, 8,* 311–317.

McDonald, C. J., Hui, S. L., Smith, D. M., Tierney, W. M., Cohen, S. J., Weinberger, M., & McCabe, G. P. (1984). Reminders to physicians from an introspective computer medical record. A two-year randomized trial. *Annals of Internal Medicine, 100,* 130–138.

Medicare and Medicaid Programs (1999). Reporting outcome and assessment information set (OASIS) data as part of the conditions of participation for home health agencies and comprehensive assessment and use of the OASIS as part of the conditions of participation for home health agencies. Final Rule. *Federal Register, 64*(15) (1999) (to be codified at 42 C.F.R. Parts 484 and 488).

Noone, C., Cavanaugh, J., & McKillip, C. (1995). Computerized documentation in home health. *Journal of Nursing Administration, 25*(1), 67–69.

Quigley, P., Mathis, A., & Nodhturft, V. (1994). Improving clinical documentation quality. *Nursing Care Quality, 8*(4), 66–73.

Rowland, H. S., & Rowland, B. L. (1997). *Nursing administration handbook.* Frederick, MD: Aspen Publishers.

Sweeney, M. A., & Skiba, D. (1995). Combining telecommunications and interactive multimedia health information on the electronic superhighway. *Medinfo, 8,* 1524–1527.

Tan, J. K. H. (1995). *Health management information systems: Theories, methods, and applications.* Gaithersburg, MD: Aspen.

Chapter 8

Patient Care Applications

Kristen S. Montgomery

The purpose of this chapter is to highlight some of the current models for integrating Internet applications into the patient care area, the strengths and weaknesses of these approaches, practical considerations, necessary resources, and future directions for using the Internet to improve patient care. Significant research in the area is highlighted.

APPLICATIONS TO PATIENT CARE

Patient Teaching

Patient teaching is a fundamental nursing activity. Almost every nurse-patient encounter includes some type of teaching activity. Nurses teach patients about their illnesses, surgery, risk factors, and how to stay healthy. Nurses also provide information on what to expect during a procedure and how it will be performed. Patients and families often seek out the nurse to answer their health care questions and to seek advice. While patient education is common in every conceivable area of practice, patient teaching is a nursing activity that may be taken for granted or omitted completely when time and other constraints interfere with adequate teaching. Transfer of knowledge from professional to consumer can be enhanced with the use of the Internet. *Enhanced* should be stressed, because the Internet, as discussed within this chapter, is not meant to replace the nurse or face-to-face contact with the nurse.

Several authors have described beginning, exploratory ways in which the Internet can be used to assist with patient education. For example, Burrows, Moore, and Lemkau (2001) described the development of a "rehabilitation prototype of a point-of-care, team-based information system (PoinTIS)" that is used for provider and patient education regarding spinal cord and traumatic brain injury. Content is disseminated via the Internet at the site where care is needed. A similar program was described by Sery-Ble, Taffe, Clarke, and Dorman (2001), in which intensive care nurses could access educational information at intranet stations throughout their unit. The authors found that their Web-based teaching tool was an effective way to train ICU nurses, and nurses who participated in this study reported that the teaching tool was easy to use and an effective way to communicate information. Programs such as these would be particularly convenient if they were available at the patient's bedside for patient and family teaching.

It has been suggested that the Internet can also be useful for accomplishing preoperative teaching for patients undergoing surgical procedures, and Klingner (2001) described the development of an intranet Web site to use as a patient and family teaching tool. The tool, known as "helping hands," consists of preprepared patient and family education sheets (pediatric focused) in the following categories: diseases and conditions, child care/safety/health information, procedures, medications, and nutrition. Any nurse in the facility can access these pages via the system-based intranet (Klingner, 2001). Education sheets are in print-ready format and can be given to patients and their families in preparation for discharge.

In an effort to determine if the Internet could also be a useful teaching tool for elders, Leaffer and Gonda (2000) conducted a study to evaluate whether Internet instruction would assist senior citizens in assuming an active role in their health care. One hundred individuals participated in the study, most of whom had a college education. The authors found that participants' confidence in using a computer was increased and that many later shared the health information they located with their health care providers (Leaffer & Gonda, 2000). Ninety days after the original training, 66% of the study participants continued to use the Internet for health-related searches. Approximately two-thirds of individuals who continued to search for health information reported that they continued to communicate with their health care provider regarding the information they found on the Internet. While this was only a pilot study with 100 participants, there are potential future applications for patient teaching, and the authors reported that more than half of those individuals who shared their findings with their health care provider were more satisfied with their care (Leaffer & Gonda, 2000). A book by Fitzpatrick, Romano, and Chasek (2001) provides a selection of consumer health Web sites suitable for patient use.

These examples represent only a few of the possibilities for using the Internet to help educate patients. In the years to come, one can expect increased use of the Internet in this capacity. As technology and Internet use continues to expand, it is likely patient education using the Internet will also expand. Further potential applications include Internet stations in every patient room, the availability of support staff to assist patients with Internet use, and Internet competent nursing staff that conduct patient teaching with the use of the Internet right at the patient's bedside.

Counseling and Support

Patient counseling regarding health and illness and patient support are additional areas in which the Internet can be utilized to improve patient care. Several authors have described the use of the Internet for patient monitoring and support, and for condition-specific support groups. For example, Biermann, Dietrich, and Standl (2000) described the use of an Internet-based monitoring system for diabetic patients to remain in contact with their health care providers. This system allows patients to report blood glucose levels and receive feedback regarding optimal blood glucose control. Biermann and colleagues conducted a prospective randomized trial with 46 patients and found that use of this system resulted in cost and time savings for both patients and health care institutions, though metabolic control did not significantly differ between those who were in the experimental and control (conventional management) groups. Complementary to this system, Kidd (2001) noted that e-mailing patients lab results may be the wave of the future.

In addition to patient physiological monitoring, the Internet can be a useful medium for emotional support networks. Hanson, Tetley, and Shewan (2000) described the use of a multimedia program to maintain the autonomy, independence, and quality of life of frail older and disabled persons and their family caregivers. Their program, ACTION (Assisting Carers using Telematic Interventions to meet Older persons' Needs), contained two parts: planning ahead and break from caring. As part of the program, participants were able to dialogue with others to meet their support needs and to obtain information to assist with decision-making.

White and Dorman (2000) described the use of an Internet mailgroup as a way to provide support to caregivers of Alzheimer's disease patients. They noted that the Internet removed several of the barriers to support group attendance that were commonly faced by the caregivers. These barriers included time constraints, geographic location, and the need for a substitute caregiver. The authors noted that benefits to the Internet-based support group included opportunities to interact with other caregivers regarding issues of guidance, information seeking, and encouragement (White & Dorman, 2000).

Walsh-Burke and Marcusen (1999) described the use of a self-advocacy training program for individuals recently diagnosed with cancer. Their program was administered by audiotape and the Internet and was developed after the completion of a study that revealed that fewer than half of the cancer patient participants (n = 565) were able to communicate their needs effectively or had the skills necessary to make decisions and negotiate with health care providers, despite the fact that the majority of participants were highly educated. Participants' ages ranged from 30 to 60. Preliminary data from pilot work with the program has revealed that the program was effective in addressing the self-advocacy skills of communication, information seeking, problem solving, decision-making, and negotiation. The authors note that the program is currently being revised to include additional groups such as older adults and pediatric patients and their families (Walsh-Burke & Marcusen, 1999).

Health Promotion

Another fruitful area for the expansion of Internet use in the patient care setting is health promotion. Health promotion activities can be divided into three main areas: primary, secondary, and tertiary, all of which are appropriate for Internet-based interventions to promote health. According to McEwen (1998) the following definitions can be used for prevention efforts: primary prevention includes activities that are directed toward preventing the occurrence of a problem or disease, secondary prevention includes activities that are aimed at early detection of disease and prompt intervention, and tertiary prevention includes limitation of disability and restoration of health, if possible, during advanced disease states. Internet-based applications for each level of prevention are discussed below.

Primary prevention consists of general health promotion, such as getting enough rest, eating well, and exercise, as well as specific protections, such as immunization and water purification (McEwen, 1998). One use of the Internet in primary prevention efforts was identified by Helwig, Lovelle, Guse, and Gottlieb (1999) who reported on use of the Internet by patients waiting for appointments in an outpatient setting. Additionally, in the area of maternal-newborn health, one new wave of the future for promoting healthy attachment between mothers and their newborns is the use of "cyber nurseries." Cyber nurseries are a free service provided by many hospitals that feature pictures of the new family member for others to view via the Internet (McCartney, 1999). In the outpatient setting, Kidd (2001) noted that e-mail reminders and follow-up may be useful to remind patients of appointments or other health promotion activities.

Secondary prevention includes activities like blood pressure screening and mammograms (McEwen, 1998). While these procedures cannot yet be done via the Internet, the Internet can be a useful medium to teach patients about these procedures, schedule appointments for the procedure, and e-mail reminders concerning the procedures. E-mail reminders of a scheduled appointment are important, but even more crucial are reminders for follow-up and routine yearly exams (e.g., physical, mammogram, Pap smears, etc.).

Health promotion at the tertiary level can also be enhanced by Internet integration. Goran and Stanford (2001) have developed "care teams" that work in collaboration with physicians to implement home monitoring for those in need of such services. Care teams monitor vital signs and retrieve patient information via the Internet. The care team concept is likely to be particularly useful for homebound elders or those who need frequent monitoring to maintain their current state of health.

Entertainment

In both the inpatient and outpatient settings, Internet access can also be utilized to decrease boredom among patients who must remain hospitalized. In addition to accessing health information on the Internet, the Internet is also a rich source for entertainment, particularly for adolescents. Many Web sites contain games that can be downloaded, and players can compete against others via the Internet. Although knowledge can be gained during Internet searching activities, the Internet can also provide a source of distraction for patients who are recovering from an illness or surgical procedure.

STRENGTHS AND WEAKNESSES

Many advantages are possible through use of the Internet in the patient care setting. Ease of access to information, instant searching capabilities, and a very comprehensive resource are but a few. While the Internet presents many interesting opportunities for improving patient care, there are precautions for its use as well. Individuals accessing the Internet must remain constantly aware of false information, since there are few regulations for content that is posted on a Web site. It is important for both consumers and health care providers to be aware that inaccurate information exists. Efforts are underway to tackle this problem; however, no system is yet perfect. Some examples of mechanisms that are in place include the Hon Code for adhering to principles of honesty while posting on the Internet. The Better Business Bureau also offers a symbol of certification for sites that maintain high business standards.

Another potential concern regarding use of the Internet in patient care settings is confidentiality. Patients and providers must be careful to ensure that personal information is not inappropriately released via the Internet. This is particularly important for patients who may not realize the potential dangers of the Internet. It is not uncommon for a specific site to require a user to register before being able to access the Web site. While registration procedures vary, often a user is prompted to enter their real name (as opposed to their user name or e-mail ID) and address. If they later enter information about their health care condition they are searching for, the two may be linked. The potential for harm with this scenario is considerable. For example, the person may be bombarded with both e-mail and postal mail regarding their condition and may receive information about "miracle cures" and other false promises. Optimistically, this bombardment constitutes a minor irritation. Pessimistically, an individual may actually try one of these "miracle cures" and may experience not only bodily harm but also the loss of the funds used to pay for the bogus treatment. Even worse, the potential exists for this information to be stored or accessed by individuals that should not have access to such private information, and the potential also exists for an overly cost-conscious insurance company to later use such information against an individual.

In addition to the legal and ethical issues mentioned above, there is the potential that some health care providers or institutions may try to use the Internet to replace nurses in certain capacities (such as patient teaching) or to decrease nurse-staffing numbers believing that the Internet can replace the need for professional staff. Another potential danger is that alternate health care providers may be expected to assume tasks that have traditionally been seen as nursing care, citing that assistive personnel are able to assume these roles with the aid of Internet technology. A final concern is that some nursing staff themselves may become too dependent on the Internet and rely on it to perform their jobs, rather than to assist them with their jobs, as has been the case with other high technology devices (e.g., critical care monitors, electronic fetal monitoring).

Although cyber nurseries are a wonderful way to help integrate the new family member, caution is warranted in terms of maintaining privacy and confidential information. The potential exists that unscrupulous individuals could access this information and harm could come to the family in the form of infant abduction from either the hospital or the home, or bombardment with offers of services and products. Most organizations have the new mother sign a consent form prior to the newborn's photo being added to the Web site (McCartney, 1999). Additionally, some facilities require a password for access or do not post the photo until after the mother and newborn are discharged (McCartney, 1999).

PRACTICAL CONSIDERATIONS AND NECESSARY RESOURCES

While there are many potential applications of the Internet to enhance patient care, there are practical considerations and resources that are necessary to make Internet-based nursing practice a reality. Organizations in which nurses practice, namely acute care facilities, will need to invest the time and resources necessary to make Internet access available on all patient units and at the patient's bedside. In addition to the physical plant resources, nurses themselves will need to take responsibility for obtaining Internet navigation skills. While employers might be willing to assume part of this burden, individual nurses, too, must assume some responsibility for integrating the Internet into patient care environments if success is to be achieved. Fortunately, most of the technology necessary to make Internet-based practice a reality has already been developed (Simpson, 2000). Our future efforts should now focus on implementation.

FUTURE DIRECTIONS

One aspect of the not so distant future is the widespread use of hand-held computers with Internet access. Wood (2001) notes that "Intelligent, autonomous software agents that guide the patient through the continuum of care will extend the reach of health care providers to all places at all times" (p. 67). Hand-held Internet access devices have a wide range of utility for nurses practicing in community health and home care settings. In addition, patients who own a hand-held device can easily bookmark Web sites that are recommended by health care providers during routine or illness-related visits. Instant bookmarking and use of the patient's own hand-held computer can facilitate use and simplify the process for all involved. Hand-held computers with Internet access are one wave of the future that is certain to have an enormous impact. While the Internet is permeating many aspects of the health care arena, the hand-held system will continue to further revolutionize health care.

In addition, nursing informatics content must be more fully integrated into the nursing educational system (Uhlenhopp, Fliedner, Morris, & Van Boxtel, 1998). There are several programs available at the Master's level that focus solely on nursing informatics, and several undergraduate programs have added informatics content to the standard curriculum. However, the integration of basic informatics content needs to be implemented more broadly so that all nurses have a basic understanding of informatics. A broad exposure to informatics during the educational process will help to ensure that nurses have the skills necessary to maintain current practice and improve patient care in all settings (Leaffer & Gonda, 2000).

SUMMARY

Many potential applications exist for improving patient care by using the Internet as part of nursing activities. Use of the Internet can significantly impact many areas of patient care. Thus far the predominant applications have been in patient teaching, patient counseling and support, health promotion, and entertainment. Many additional applications are potentially available.

The hand-held computer with portable Internet access is likely to revolutionize health care. Nurses and health care institutions will both need to assume partial responsibility for effective and efficient use of the Internet to enhance patient care. Appropriately wiring the physical plant and integration of informatics content into the nursing curricula are the first steps to achieve this goal.

REFERENCES

Biermann, E., Dietrich, W., & Standl, E. (2000). Telecare of diabetic patients with intensified insulin therapy. A randomized clinical trial. *Studies in Health Technology and Informatics, 77*, 327–332.

Burrows, S. C., Moore, K. M., & Lemkau, H. L. (2001). Creating a Web-accessible, point-of-care, team-based information system (PoinTIS): The librarian as publisher. *Bulletin of the Medical Librarians Association, 89*, 154–164.

Fitzpatrick, J. J., Romano, C., & Chasek, R. (Eds.). (2001). *The nurses' guide to consumer health Web sites.* New York: Springer Publishing Co.

Goran, M. J., & Stanford, J. (2001). E-health: Restructuring care delivery in the Internet age. *Journal of Healthcare Informatics Management, 15*, 3–12.

Hanson, E. J., Tetley, J., & Shewan, J. (2000). Supporting family carers using interactive multimedia. *British Journal of Nursing, 9*, 713–719.

Helwig, A. L., Lovelle, A., Guse, C. E., & Gottieb, M. S. (1999). An office-based Internet patient education system: A pilot study. *Journal of Family Practice, 48*, 123–127.

Kidd, M. (2001). General practice on the Internet. *Australian Family Physician, 30*, 359–361.

Klingner, A. (2001). Helping hands for nursing staff. *Nursing News, 7*(2), 5.

Leaffer, T., & Gonda, B. (2000). The Internet: An underutilized tool in patient education. *Computers in Nursing, 18*, 47–52.

McCartney, P. R. (1999). Confidentiality and privacy with discussion lists and "cyber nurseries." *MCN: The American Journal of Maternal Child Nursing, 24*, 263.

McEwen, M. (1998). *Community-based nursing: An introduction.* Philadelphia: W. B. Saunders.

Sery-Ble, O. R., Taffe, E. R., Clarke, A. W., & Dorman, T. (2001). Use of and satisfaction with a browser-based nurse teaching tool in a surgical intensive care unit. *Computers in Nursing, 19*, 82–86.

Simpson, R. L. (2000). The role of IT in caring for the chronically ill. *Nursing Administration Quarterly, 24*, 82–85.

Uhlenhopp, M. B., Fliedner, M. C., Morris, P., & Van Boxtel, T. (1998). A global perspective on nurses' Internet access and information utilization. *Oncology Nursing Forum, 25*(10, Suppl.), 27–32.

Walsh-Burke, K., & Marcusen, C. (1999). Self-advocacy training for cancer survivors. The cancer survival toolbox. *Cancer Practice, 7*, 297–301.

White, M. H., & Dorman, S. M. (2000). Online support for caregivers. Analysis of an Internet Alzheimer mailgroup. *Computers in Nursing, 18*, 168–176.

Wood, G. M. (2001). Emerging technologies in health care and the patient encounter of the future. *Management and Care Interface, 14*(3), 67–70.

Chapter 9

Security Concerns in Clinical Settings

Mary L. McHugh

I n previous chapters, the various benefits of using the Internet in clinical practice were discussed. Some precautions are warranted, however. These can be grouped into dangers from staff, from strangers, and from the "open window" that e-mail systems inadvertently create. Most of these dangers can be eliminated or greatly reduced through carefully prepared and enforced policies about passwords and computer use. Others can be controlled through software and hardware devices. System security is one of the most difficult—and perhaps the most important—part of the information technology (IT) manager's job. But security cannot be only the IT manager's job. What is important to teach the hospital's staff and management is that system security is everybody's job. The Internet can be a tremendously valuable source of information. It can also be the vehicle through which the hospital's information system (HIS) is damaged or destroyed. System security requires another complete system, including software, hardware, policies, and an educated and aware workforce. In this chapter, the sources of danger to the HIS and its data are identified along with methods for protecting against each danger.

SOURCES OF DANGER

Viruses and Worms

The Internet is a window to the outside world. Nurses may use that window to access a wealth of information, but unfortunately, that window can also make the system vulnerable to viruses and worms. Almost everyone has heard about the damage that computer viruses can do to an institution's database. A specialized form of virus called a "worm" can also enter through e-mail windows and cause considerable damage.

A *computer virus* is a piece of programming code attached to some innocuous item of mail or other program and transmitted in some way by the virus programmer. A few viruses (like the well-known "Happy Birthday" virus) have been designed to just send silly messages and not to do any damage to the recipient's files or programs. Innocuous viruses are the exception. Most other viruses are designed to do two things. First, they typically are designed to spread—usually by attaching to the recipient's e-mail system and automatically sending themselves to every other person listed in the recipient's e-mail address book. Second, they typically damage the recipients programs, data files, or system files. Some cause so much damage that the only way to recover is to reformat the hard drive, thus losing all programs, data, and information on the hard drive.

Computer worms can have two meanings in cyberspeech. The "good" meaning of worm is a form of permanent, high-density storage called *write once, read many* disk. The "bad" meaning of worm is a specialized form of computer virus that tends not to do immediate damage to the hard drive. Rather, it continually replicates itself and takes up increasing amounts of space on the hard drive until the entire hard drive is filled up. Then it begins to overwrite parts of data and program files. In some cases, it is designed to immediately start overwriting files so that the files become riddled with "holes," almost as if a real worm were eating its way through the user's programs and data files. Worms can be very hard to discover because they often cause damage so subtly that it is weeks or even months before the user realizes that the system has a serious problem. It can take the IS experts quite a while to correctly diagnose the problem and then clean the system—not to mention finding all other infected systems and cleaning up that damage too. Typical effects of a worm include the system speed becoming noticeably compromised, programs that run, but with certain features not working, or formerly good data files suddenly having parts damaged. Ultimately, if not stopped, the worm damages everything.

Damage From Viruses and Worms

Viruses and worms typically get into a computer system through e-mail. Unfortunately, some of the very features that make e-mail most useful also create vulnerabilities for the systems that allow e-mail in. The ability to attach programs and documents to e-mail is one of the most important facilities for users. Clinicians may want to send each other clinical care protocols for patients with rare diseases, or they may want to share parts of a newly written procedure or other documents that can save the recipient much time in developing or typing the document. Loss of the ability to send e-mail attachments would certainly reduce the value of e-mail tremendously. E-mail attachments are not easily scanned by the server's antivirus software, however, and thus are an attractive target for malicious virus programmers. Due to the danger of viruses, many university systems now ban all e-mail with attachments that are executable programs. The following file extensions on attachments are cause for great concern (and many are banned by university mail server systems): .EXE, .COM, .SYS, .OVL, .PRG, and .MNU. A virus is a program, and thus it needs an executable file name. Sadly, many people need to send programs to each other, and the virus programmers have destroyed that option for thousands of innocent users.

In addition to e-mail, viruses can get into systems by diskettes containing game programs purchased through Internet advertisers and, worse, programs directly downloaded from the Internet through discussion boards and Internet bulletin boards. The best advice is NEVER download an executable program from the Internet. Or if a program file must be downloaded, download it onto a diskette, zip drive, or other storage medium that can be isolated from the HIS. A virus detection program can then be executed on the disk or zip drive prior to opening the program. Some facilities keep a PC that is not connected in any way to the rest of the HIS for the purpose of downloading and using potentially infected programs. That way, if the program is infected, it may cause damage to the isolated computer, but not to the entire HIS. This is extremely similar to quarantining a person infected with a highly contagious disease. In both cases, an effective quarantine keeps the infection from spreading beyond the individual person or computer.

At the time of this printing, it is still considered fairly safe to download and print documents and pages from the Internet (so long as copyright laws are respected), but downloading games and other executable programs is extremely risky. Because most people enjoy computer games, it is not unusual for staff to download games during slow work times. Unfortunately, many hospital computer systems have become infected with computer viruses from this kind of activity. The most serious concern with having Internet access on a clinical unit is that a virus could enter the HIS through the Internet and damage or compromise the programs and confidential data in the hospital's database.

A virus can damage not only the recipient's computer, but also any other computer linked to the computer that first received the virus. As a result, a whole hospital information system could be irreparably damaged from a virus that entered via an e-mail message to a desktop computer in the nurses' station. If the timing is particularly bad—for example, the virus enters just before a major system backup procedure—the virus might end up incorporated into the backup storage medium. In this instance, often the whole HIS hard drive has to be erased and reloaded to rid the system of the virus. Otherwise, backup drives might continue to reinfect the computer until the system administrator discovers all instances of the virus and destroys them. At least once or twice a year, most major computer facilities have to take the whole system down for a day or two to try and clean out a virus that has infected hundreds of the PCs in a system. Unfortunately, it is not terribly unusual for one or two office computers to be missed in the general clean up. When these users start their system, the entire computer system may get reinfected. Another day or two can be lost as the IS employees try to remove the virus a second time. To the extent that a hospital has its patient charts, administrative and billing records, and payroll and other critical systems on the computer that gets infected, a virus could cause such disruption that patient care becomes adversely affected.

Computer Spam

The general meaning of "spam" in the world of e-mail is any unsolicited and unwanted e-mail. More specifically, when an unwanted item of e-mail is sent repeatedly so that the user's mailbox is literally filled up with repetitive and unwanted messages, the recipient is said to have been "spammed." Some programs have been written to repeatedly replicate an e-mail message and send it in an infinite loop to all members of a facility's address book. This is called "spamming."

What this means is that some e-mail message goes to a recipient's mailbox. When the recipient opens the e-mail, it attaches to the recipient's address book and sends itself to every person listed. Unfortunately, it doesn't send just one copy. It continues to send the same message repeatedly—in an infinite loop.* Such a program has no end point. It keeps resending the same e-mail to everybody until the e-mail system becomes overwhelmed and crashes. It may also end if the amount of allocated storage space for e-mail is exceeded. (Both outgoing and incoming e-mails have to be stored on the server until deleted.) When the user's e-mail box is filled with spam, the user can receive no legitimate e-mail. It often takes hours to delete all the spam from both the inbox and outbox.

Hackers

The word "hackers" originally meant someone who was very interested in personal computers and explored the capabilities of these machines. Over time, however, the word has come to have a more sinister meaning. Today, most people think of a hacker as a person who directly breaks into other people's computers for the purpose of stealing private information or causing damage to files and programs. A virus is a type of time bomb. The virus programmer is not personally using the recipient's computer when the damage is done. A hacker gains entry into private computers by using the Internet as a pathway. The portal of entry is usually a password. The problem is that many people fail to protect their passwords.

Most hospitals have strict rules about how passwords are to be protected, and staff are not to reveal their personal passwords to anyone—not even to other staff members. However, human nature being what it is, people often are extraordinarily careless with passwords. Passwords are hard for many people to remember. In many installations, the IS personnel change the passwords every 3 months or so, which can contribute to increased difficulty remembering a password. Assignment of nonsense passwords composed of a random mixture of letters and numbers can further contribute to this problem. When a password is forgotten, it can be time consuming to obtain from the IS department. Worse, night shift IS people are often available only by pager and they get very angry at being roused out of bed for a forgotten

---

*An infinite loop means the program orders a command to be carried out, but at the end, it doesn't tell the computer to stop and go back to the user for a new command. Instead, it orders the computer to go back to the beginning of the command sequence and start executing the same command again. When the command is to send an e-mail message to everybody in the address book, it doesn't take long for thousands of e-mail messages to be generated.

password. Nurses just want to perform their patient care duties. Given health care's increasing dependency on computers and a normal human's inability to remember a constantly changed, nonsense password, the easiest way to function is to compromise password security.

To be sure passwords are available to legitimate users, nurses have to write them down somewhere. That somewhere is often a fairly public place in the unit. The author has seen the whole list of staff passwords neatly typed and taped to the side of the computer at the nurses' station. This makes them convenient for any casual passerby to inspect—and later use to hack into the hospital's computer. In one case, a hacker saw the list taped to the computer, took the list and made a copy in the bathroom, and then retaped it to the computer—all without anyone in the unit noticing anything was amiss. Later, the entire list appeared on a hacker bulletin board on the Internet, and potentially thousands of hackers had access to the passwords. Other passwords have been compromised when nurses taped them to their own computer at home. Friends of teenage children have used the passwords to hack into the hospital's computer "for fun." These postings of passwords are strictly against policy. But the problem here is really not a "bad nurses" problem, it is a system design problem. The IS department has designed a security system that few humans can implement safely and consistently over time. Therefore, people have to find ways to override the protection system if they are to do their primary job—in the nurse's case patient care. The only real solution is to design a people-friendly security system. How to do that will be addressed in the section on how to overcome dangers.

Inadvertent Security Lapses

Offering Internet access on the patient care unit often happens through the same PC that the staff uses to access the entire HIS. Staff may inadvertently infect the system with viruses by unwise downloading, by opening e-mail with infected attachments, and by bringing infected diskettes from home and using them on the hospital computers without first running them through an antivirus program. Staff may leave their passwords in places that hackers can find them. Staff may give each other their passwords for convenience. This often happens when one nurse's patient load suddenly gets to be too much because a patient deteriorated unexpectedly—perhaps even coded—or the nurse had to take an admission or two, or perhaps another nurse whose load was light just offered to help. One way nurses sometimes help each other is to chart vital signs and other information. It is not rare for a busy nurse to share a private password with another nurse so that nurse can chart for her. Their purpose is not to violate security. Nurses are merely trying to give the best possible patient care. They often feel that the computers should have been designed and set up to promote that goal, not to serve as a barrier to top-quality and efficient patient care. When the computer security system interferes with their real work, it is no wonder nurses bypass the security protocols.

Lack of Privacy

Although some might not recognize this as a danger, every employee needs to understand that their use of the Internet on an office computer is not private. Somehow, most people have assumed that since it is illegal for an employer to open any U.S. Postal Service mail addressed to an employee, that their e-mail is equally protected. It is not! A case pertaining to an employer firing an employee based on something contained in an e-mail the employee sent from his work computer was pursued all the way to the U.S. Supreme Court. The court decided in the employer's favor. The reasoning is that the company computers all belong to the employer. The employer is entitled to use, look at, keep or destroy its property in any way it chooses. Unless the employer explicitly gives employees the right to use that computer (including the employee's company e-mail account) privately, there is no right to privacy. Your employer is quite capable of reading any e-mail without even entering your office computer.

E-mail.   E-mail is stored on the company Internet server, and any system administrator or programmer can look at all e-mail stored on the server. In fact, programs can be written to scan all e-mail and retrieve and print any with certain specified characters or character strings. An employer could scan for vulgar words or for his/her own name. If an employee sent out an e-mail complaining about how incompetent, unfair, or unattractive the boss is, the boss has every right to read that e-mail. And certainly the boss has the right to discover if employees are using company computers to compromise confidential data, reports, or other information. The employer can use the e-mail

as evidence of misconduct in support of an action to involuntarily terminate the employee. E-mail is actually much better evidence of misconduct than the testimony of other employees or managers about what
the terminated employee did or said. E-mail is a written document—the
strongest kind of evidence possible.

Inappropriate Internet sites. Most companies have policies that
company computers cannot be used to visit pornographic sites, and
indeed, should be used only to visit business-related Internet sites.
Employees should be aware that the computer keeps a log of all Internet
sites visited, and that the IS department can write programs that provide
a list by individual password of all sites visited. Thus, employees can
find themselves in disciplinary difficulty for using the company Internet
account to visit sexually explicit sites, auction sites, and other sites
that have no relevance to work. There is no assumption of privacy for
use of company computers to "surf the Net."

METHODS TO PROTECT AGAINST THE DANGERS
OF THE INTERNET

Policy Protections

The most basic protection a hospital must have is to write policies
pertaining to staff behavior. The policies must be taught during orientation, reviewed yearly, and enforced vigorously. In some hospitals, the
penalty for compromising a password is suspension for the first violation, and termination for the second. People will forget policies, so they
must be reminded frequently. Unit managers must be asked to enforce
the computer security policies and to remind their staff members of
the danger to the entire system—and, of course, to patient confidentiality—of any lapses in staff behavior with respect to computer security.

Password security policies. The most important policy pertaining
to computer system security is the policy demanding that people keep
their personal passwords secret. If passwords are used, a two-pass-
word sequence should be implemented. The first password is often
called a "user identifier" (Userid). It tells the computer the category of
employee who is signing on, and is typically linked to a table of privi-

leges. The table of privileges identifies what data and programs that user can access. All nurses in a particular unit may have the same Userid. Or all members of the nursing department may share one Userid. The second level password is the individual's personal password. Each nurse receives a personal password so the computer knows who is signing on whenever that password is used. Userids are not very secret. Typically, a fairly large number of people share a single Userid. However, the personal password is supposed to be known only to the individual who owns that password and perhaps to the system administrator. When people reveal their passwords to others—even to coworkers, nobody can be really sure who signed on using that password. This makes it difficult to use the password as a legal signature (which is important in health records). Worse, it makes protecting the confidentiality of private health records impossible. Therefore, strict policies about keeping one's password secret are an important part of the system security plan.

The critical fact is that violations of password security are the behavioral norm in a hospital unless action is taken to stop the behavior. The staff are not computer professionals. Thus, most staff have little understanding of the dangers of computer security violations. In addition, password security violations are quick, easy, and very convenient. They often help nurses carry out the patient care part of their jobs more easily and more efficiently. This constellation of circumstances makes password violations inevitable unless something is done to ensure that people fear the consequences much more than they value the convenience.

Typically, password policies are short and to the point. First, everyone is to keep his or her password strictly secret. Passwords are not to be revealed to anyone else—not to a coworker, unit manager, and certainly not to patients, visitors, or anyone at home. Second, the consequences of violating the password security policy must be explicit and severe. In many cases, the first violation will result in a suspension (which is often a third-level disciplinary action). Password protection (and physical violence) policies are atypical because most disciplinary policies start with a verbal warning, progress to a written warning, and then to actual disciplinary action. This is considered insufficient for password security. The opinion is that staff must be made to understand that *any* violations of password security are extremely serious and will not be tolerated. The policy may even state that violations of password security are considered flagrant violations of patient confidentiality and will be met with immediate and severe disciplinary action. If a second violation occurs, the disciplinary action should be immediate termination.

The suggested consequences are obviously severe. The purpose is to shock people into protecting their passwords. Creating a strong emotional reaction to password violations has been found to be the only way to impress upon staff the need to maintain password security. Management must understand that password violations are easy, convenient, and very common. Maintaining security is difficult, inconvenient, and annoying to the staff—especially when passwords are nonsensical and changed often. Management is demanding that staff do something that makes their job harder. To gain compliance, the consequences must be so terrible that it is seen as more desirable to live with the inconvenience than to violate security.

If the hospital is to have any control over access to its data and programs, it has to make sure passwords are kept extremely secure. Mild disciplinary actions will not impel staff to forego password violations. If people think that the consequences are tolerable, and especially if they do not expect to get caught because "everybody is doing it," passwords will quickly become an open, public portal into the hospital's confidential data. A suspension or termination of someone who "only gave someone else her password" will create the emotional shock necessary to force people to comply with the policy. It will personalize the action because every other staff member will relate to the error and the consequence. And the story will be spread far and wide among the staff that someone got fired because she compromised her password.

Hardware and Software Protections

In some situations, the IS department can provide security with computer hardware or software. If this approach can be used to bypass the need for human compliance with hated policies, much time, effort, and problems with staff-management relations might be saved. Password security systems are cheap for the hospital, but as discussed, they are not very effective. They require a huge investment in management time to teach staff about the importance of security and the consequences for security violations. And management must be ever vigilant about such violations. In some states, labor judges will not allow management to enforce consequences for policy violations unless every violation is met with the same punishment. Management may be extremely reluctant to terminate a registered nurse for a security violation in an era characterized by severe nursing shortages. In some units, terminating a nurse who cannot be quickly replaced could result in the need to close beds and lose business. If computer-based solutions can be found so that password security becomes unnecessary, much time, effort, and emotional distress could be saved.

Physical recognition devices.   The first hardware that can be used for system security involves physical recognition technology. Passwords were designed so that the system could discriminate between people who were authorized to access the system and those who have no right to enter the system. For many years, the owners of systems in which security was a prime concern have recognized that password security is ineffective.

The defense department is one key player in the area of secure systems. They have long used physical recognition technology to keep unauthorized users out of their systems. The most common physical recognition systems use finger, retinal, and palm prints to identify legitimate users. The price of this technology is initially much higher than using password security. However, over time, it is less expensive than paying the numerous people necessary to enforce password security policies. Fingerprint recognition hardware today costs less than $1,000 per machine (originally, it was about $20,000 per machine). When a new employee is hired, the fingerprint is recorded in the system, along with the access privileges of that employee. Each time the employee wants to access the computer, the finger is simply placed in a print reader device and system recognition allows the employee to access the system. It is physically impossible for the average hacker to overcome that protection device. Such passive security devices save staff a lot of time, emotion, and supervision effort. They are also much more secure.

Antivirus protection programs.   Several companies have developed and marketed software designed to detect viruses and worms, and to block them before they can infect the system. The two most popular products in this line include the Norton and McAfee antivirus programs (both are copyrighted). Both products have Web sites designed to let product purchasers update their products, and they provide lots of helpful information about how to keep a system clean and free of viruses. Every computer should have an antivirus protection program.

Isolated Internet computers.   One of the safest ways to ensure that unauthorized persons cannot gain access to the hospital's information system is to keep that data in computers that are isolated from all outside contact. The only way a hacker can gain access to a computer system is through the lines from the computer to outside networks. These lines might be phone lines (modem linkup), cable modem, DSL lines, and T-lines, but all lines to the outside world function as a door into the HIS. Even when that door has a fairly secure lock, there is a danger of a "thief" figuring out how to break open that lock. If, however, there is no door, then breaking in cannot happen through the Internet linkages. In this model, all hospital computers in the network are directly wired to each other. There is no outside line linked into the hospital's computer network. Therefore, the only way viruses can get into the system is through diskettes or CD-ROMs brought into the facility, or if an internal person loads a destructive program directly into the system. Some facilities have computers with no CD-ROM or diskette drive. That approach virtually eliminates accidental introduction of viruses into the system. It also eliminates most opportunity for employees to make illicit copies of confidential data, unless they make illicit printouts. The problem with this approach, of course, is that without special hardware it eliminates all access to the benefits of the Internet.

One way to have the Internet available when the hospital has a closed intranet system is to have a second, special computer located in each unit. The second computer is linked to the Internet through a phone line and modem, but has no link to the HIS. A modem is a fairly slow connection, but if that Internet computer is not linked in any way to the hospital's computer, then viruses and hackers can not use that computer or the Internet as a link into the HIS. They can still damage the unit's isolated Internet computer, but the damage is limited to that machine alone. Internet-only computers can be extremely cheap. They do not need all the power of Microsoft's Windows® operating system. A very simple, cheap operating system, the Netscape browser, a modem or other linkage hardware, and connection software are all that is needed to have full access to the Internet. In fact, the hospital could offer high-speed Internet access on such machines with DSL, cable modem, or T1/T2 lines fairly inexpensively. Such single-purpose machines can cost less than $500. Purchased in bulk so that each hospital unit can have one will bring the price even lower. If the computer becomes infected despite antivirus software, it is a fairly simple procedure for the IS support people to clean up the problem. They may need to reformat the hard drive to completely rid the computer of a virus. However, reloading all software for the single-purpose Internet machine would take less than an hour. Hackers may find a way to access the information on the isolated computer, but will not be able to compromise confidential patient data in the hospital's HIS since the two are not linked in any way.

Firewall. Having the HIS be entirely an intranet, that is, isolated from all outside links, has not been used much. The benefits of having the entire HIS networked through the Internet are so great that a different software protection approach has typically been adopted. Many HIS departments have installed a firewall to protect their system from problems. A firewall may be a hardware device that contains protective software, or it may be strictly a software approach. In either case, it is designed to block access to the HIS by unauthorized persons and to identify and block hidden code (which is almost always a virus) in messages or in downloads from the Internet. A firewall sits at the junction between the internal network and the link from the outside computer world into the private network.

The software in a firewall examines all traffic entering or leaving the private network to see if it meets criteria specified by the IS programmers. If an outside hacker doesn't have a legitimate Userid and password (or a recognized physical pattern from a physical recognition system), entry is blocked by the firewall. Another way firewalls often filter out unauthorized persons is to check the ID of the computer the hacker is using. As part of setting up a password or physical recognition system, the system administrators can also program the system to permit access to their system to only identified computers. When authorized users want to enter from home, part of the setup procedure involves them registering their computer's unique identifier with the firewall software.

Even with a legitimate Userid and Password, the hacker will be unsuccessful unless he or she is using the legitimate user's computer. The firewall cannot protect against misbehavior or deliberate sabotage by a legitimate user. This is why policies against revealing passwords are so important. Additionally, sabotage by terminated employees has been a serious problem for some companies. Almost anybody can have high-tech skills today. The IS department should not assume that an employee does not have well developed programming and Internet capabilities. Indeed, some of the most successful hackers in history have been high-school children.

The simple activity of terminating passwords and changing Userid codes for a department whenever an employee leaves (either voluntarily or involuntarily) is the most basic safety procedure for any competent IS department. In fact, if an employee is to leave involuntarily, it is usually a good procedure for the facility to coordinate unit management, IS security, and hospital security personnel. The procedure should be to call the IS manager as soon as the employee enters the unit manager's office to be informed of the dismissal. At that instant, the employee's password should be terminated. The employee should then be required to turn in any name tag or other ID materials, escorted to the unit to retrieve all his or her belongings and escorted by hospital security out of the building. It is much safer to give terminated employees two weeks pay free than to give them two weeks notice and risk compromise of the computer system during that time. This seems cruel because very few terminated employees will actually commit acts of sabotage. However, one disgruntled employee with some sophisticated computer skills can do millions of dollars worth of damage to a modern computer system.

There can be some real disadvantages to firewalls. Some were designed to allow the user to passively view all Internet sites that contain information, but to block all interactive sites. Such a firewall stops computer use for online continuing education (CE). CE sites have to be interactive so that the employee can be identified and can take and submit tests online. Many Internet college courses now exist and the great majority of those sites require the student to participate in a class discussion board. Firewalls that block interactive sites block Internet college courses. Some firewalls allow users to print Internet pages, but not to download anything. This can be a real problem if it forces people to retype pages of information. If that solution is deemed essential by IS, perhaps a scanner could be added to the unit Internet computer so that printed information from the Internet can be scanned in. Scanned pages cannot contain viruses. For those interested in learning more about firewalls, there is an excellent introductory article about firewalls at the following URL: *http://www.vicomsoft.com/ knowledge/reference/firewalls1.html?track=internal.*

Lack of Privacy

There is only one protection for employees against lack of privacy. Buy your own computer for home and obtain a private e-mail account. Personal resources can then be used with great care. Nothing you do on the Internet is really private. Private e-mail and Internet accounts are typically obtained through public companies that sell accounts that allow the user to access the Internet. Typically, e-mail accounts are provided as part of a package. The ISP provider can see everything you do because your commands, e-mail, and the Internet pages you access are handled through the ISP's Internet server (a special computer). Your employer would need a subpoena to access your home computer or private account e-mail. To obtain such a subpoena, the employer would need to file a civil or criminal misconduct suit and show a judge some evidence that your home computer should be made open to search and seizure. However, Internet service providers own the server and can look at anything they wish.

Unless there is a contract that limits their use of your personal information, they can use your name, address, Internet preferences, or any other information about you they can glean from your contacts in any way they wish. ISPs often have policies about pornography and might even have policies that allow them to report you to the police if they detect criminal behavior. It is important to be aware that even your private account e-mail and the Internet sites you view are stored and logged on a public server. People who use their personal computers for criminal activities have no absolute right to privacy for what they do on their home computers. The owners of Internet servers can look at anything on their machines that they wish to view. The best policy for individuals is to use an employer's computer only for legitimate business. Only send out e-mail that you are comfortable having your employer read. Visit Internet sites only if they can be directly linked to your efforts to do your job. Limit personal use of the computer to the machine you personally own and keep at home. Even for your home computer, keep in mind that somewhere ISPs keep a record of everything you do through their servers. Do not deliberately go to sites, send e-mail, or place materials on the Internet that would give you problems with a criminal defense suit in a public courtroom.

CONCLUSIONS

There are potential dangers to allowing Internet access in a patient care unit. Internet access carries with it the risk of opening the door to viruses and worms, the danger that e-mail accounts will be flooded with spam, and that staff will inadvertently let hackers in through carelessness with passwords. In addition, employees can personally compromise their jobs through unwise use of e-mail and by visiting inappropriate Internet sites while at work.

Although no protection scheme is perfect, a variety of hardware and software tools have been developed to help companies protect the confidentially and security of information systems. Policies properly written and strictly enforced can reduce incidences of employees becoming careless with passwords. Physical recognition devices can make passwords obsolete and offer a much higher degree of security for the company's information system. One approach that has been used to both provide Internet access and yet keep the HIS isolated from the dangers of the Internet is to have Internet access provided only through special, isolated computers on the unit that have no connection to the computers containing patient information. That solution has not been adopted often, because most IS managers are now implementing firewall technology to control access to their internal computer network. Firewalls create constraints and barriers that may limit the benefits of Internet use.

WEB SITE RECAP

Firewalls
http://www.vicomsoft.com/knowledge/reference/firewalls1.html?track=internal

Part II

Educational Applications

Chapter **10**

Distance Education and Web-Based Courses

Jeanne M. Novotny and Tami H. Wyatt

In a small town in rural Michigan, Jan, a 32-year-old advanced practice nurse and working mother, carries her groceries from her car
into her house. It is late afternoon and after putting her groceries
away she sits down at her computer and logs into a continuing
education class. She takes a quiz to see if she got the main points
of her last session. She then downloads a recommended reading
that impacts the care she is delivering to one of her oncology patients.
Next she gets into a chat room and asks for specific information
related to one of her patients from an expert and from other practitioners who are also enrolled in the same asynchronous continuing
education program.

Tom, a 38-year-old registered nurse with an associate degree, comes
home from an evening shift at a large medical center in Atlanta. He
has a midnight snack and logs on to his computer. He is taking a
nursing theory class from a well-known professor. This class is one
of the requirements for his baccalaureate degree. He accesses the
library collection and downloads one of the required readings. A
message comes across his computer screen from one of his classmates. This classmate lives in Alaska. The two communicate in their
virtual chat space. Although they have never met face to face, they
have become friends and plan to graduate at the same time.

These examples demonstrate how the Internet is revolutionizing
nursing education. Jan and Tom have opportunities for continuous

professional development because of the Internet and the distance education programs that are now available. These are not students who would be sitting in a traditional classroom. They are receiving a quality education that would otherwise be unavailable to them.

The purpose of this chapter is to briefly review the background of distance education, to compare and contrast traditional and Internet instruction, and to describe the questions that potential students need to ask before choosing a program of study or online continuing education offering. It is specifically directed to the registered nurse and advanced practice nurse.

Technology is providing practicing nurses and nursing students with the opportunity to learn, share information, and collaborate with colleagues throughout the world. A distance-education format will not meet the needs of all learners; however, it is ideal for the individual who is motivated, needs flexibility, and wants to maintain professional accountability through self-evaluation and ongoing education. Internet-based education is a learning option that is based on the assumption that the student will become a part of a community of learners even as they work separated from each other and their instructor. Nurses not interested in using the Internet for educational purposes also will feel its effects because technology is changing the traditional classroom in subtle and profound ways.

Degree-granting institutions and continuing education programs are facing critical challenges. It is important to understand these challenges in order to understand why Internet education will become increasingly important in the 21st century. In order to remain viable, traditional educational programs must:

- Provide first-rate leadership and instruction in rapidly developing new areas of knowledge and specialization,
- Meet the learning needs of an increasingly diverse student population,
- Hire faculty who are flexible and have the ability to incorporate research findings and technology into everyday instructional practices,
- Address political pressures for greater accountability for measurable learning results (Gifford, 1995).

Because of these challenges new ways of addressing the way we teach and how we learn are of the utmost importance. As universities, associations, private providers and others compete in the marketplace for formal and continuing professional education, increasing numbers of learners will turn to the Internet as a convenient, satisfying, and economically prudent way to save time and money to keep current in their field. Not only does the Internet deliver online classes, it also creates "virtual communities" where professionals can communicate, get current information, and conduct business on a daily basis.

HISTORICAL PERSPECTIVE

The first time a student opts for an Internet course she/he is embarking on an adventure. Nurses have a rich history of seeking the latest educational method to get the education that they need to remain current. The evolution of American educational technology is slightly different than the technology historically used in nursing education. During the early 1900s, the American visual instruction movement combined with the radio movement established innovative forms of learning (Saettler, 1990), but it was not until the late twentieth century that the nursing profession began using film/video and radio technology as a form of distance education. The concept of using communication tools that are not bound by time and space to bring education to learners far and wide began with print media and correspondence studies. This method required sending and receiving assignments via postal mail. The use of radio in education began as early as the 1920s, but little is known about the effectiveness of this medium on instruction (Saettler, 1990). Although broadcast radio was typically a format for one-way lectures or presentations (Heinich, Molenda, Russell, & Smaldino, 1999), some interactivity between faculty and students provided the first immediate feedback with distance education (Armstrong, 2000). By World War II, the use of educational radio declined with educators more interested in television technology. Television technology became popular in the 1960s when a variety of video-based initiative television systems became available. This form of broadcast uses asynchronous transfer mode (ATM) using videoconferencing equipment. Typically, programs using ATM videoconferencing equipment with televisions connect two or more classrooms to one another with an instructor in one of the locations. This technology is still popular today because of its close resemblance to the traditional classroom. Some nursing programs combine various forms of distance education modalities to attract students in far reaching places. These programs, known as external degree programs, use video/film technology, print media, videoconferencing technology, and often the Internet as a way to deliver instruction. They differ from traditional programs because the learning experience does not offer a prescribed method of learning. Instead, the learning is independent (Nichols, 1997).

Computer technology for distance education has leaped into the forefront partially because of technological advances as well as educational reform (Armstrong, Gessner, & Cooper, 2000). Writings about distance education have almost doubled from 1988 to 1991 due to the technological advances (Ely, Foley, Freeman, & Scheel, 1995). The Internet is the newest and the most versatile distance education vehicle. It has the potential to provide the best of all worlds. It incorporates multimedia and self-paced learning, and offers multiple venues for communication and connectivity (Garrison, Schardt, & Kochi, 2000). All aspects of nursing will be touched by the phenomena of the Internet and the multiple opportunities that it presents for innovative approaches to learning.

The need for degree completion, skill acquisition, continuing education, and certificate nursing education will continue to proliferate. A shift in restructured health care environments to an emphasis on primary and ambulatory care provided in clinics, community, and other settings, requires additional knowledge, skills, and expertise. Nurses seeking to remain competitive in the health care market will need the community assessment, problem solving, and clinical management skills that are taught at the baccalaureate level (Beason, 1997). Historically nursing has always been able to evolve continuously in its methods, structure, and educational approaches to meet the changing health care needs of society. Thus, the Internet is a means to meet the health care challenges of society and the profession that are both clinically relevant and educationally viable.

DIFFERENCES BETWEEN TRADITIONAL AND INTERNET INSTRUCTION

If you are a potential distance-education student, it is important to understand the differences between traditional and electronic instruction. Distance education is defined as a set of teaching and/or learning strategies to meet the learning needs of students separate from the traditional classroom setting and sometimes from the traditional roles of faculty (Reinert & Fryback, 1997).

The two basic models of distance education are synchronous and asynchronous (Table 10.1). In synchronous learning, the teacher and the student interact in real time. The use of two-way video conferencing is an example of synchronous learning. Synchronous learning decreases flexibility. It requires all students to be online, in a videoconference, or in a classroom at the same time. Asynchronous learning occurs when individuals access the educational materials independently and at times and places of their choice. Asynchronous activities allow the student to take as much time as they want to read the materials and compose responses or messages. They also allow time for reflection and result in thoughtful discussion. The use of asynchronous technology extends the reach of education to previously unserved or underserved populations as well as to those who prefer a more self-directed learning environment (Lewis, 2000). It is the most flexible and friendly way to use the Internet for formal degree programs and continuing education.

Distance learning offers new opportunities for nurses who are seeking basic or advanced degrees, certificates, or lifelong learning for professional development (Billings, Ward, & Penton-Cooper, 2001). The advantages to using the Internet are many. First, convenience and easy access are the cornerstones. The course work may be self-paced and asynchronous. The student has easy access to online libraries, databases, and learning resources. The ability to network with colleagues in specialty areas without any geographic limitations is unlimited. There are several disadvantages. The student needs a computer, modem, Internet service provider, and basic computer literacy skills (Novotny & Murley, 1999). Bandwidth and connectivity to the Internet are issues that continue to exist in Internet-based education. This is especially true for individuals who have computers with slower modems or those learners who live in communities with less capable speed connectivity. Additionally, individual learners must recognize their personal learning style and determine if Internet-based education is appropriate. The work in developing and implementing a quality distance education program occurs before students ever begin. The spirit and potential of distance education can best be realized by programs that are specifically designed and implemented on the basis of the needs of the identified population of learners for whom the program is intended.

TABLE 10.1   Asynchronous Versus Synchronous Distance Learning Methodologies via the Internet

Learning methodology	Asynchronous	Synchronous

Video	Prerecorded Webcasts, videoconference, or presentation to be viewed at student's convenience	Real-time videoconference streaming:
		  One-way videoconferencing: learner can see and hear the conference but cannot interact with the speaker
		  Two-way videoconferencing: learner can see, hear, and interact with the speaker by 1) typing responses, 2) voice and video with videoconferencing technology

Document sharing/assignments	Sending documents or assignments via e-mail, listservs, or threaded discussion or storing documents on Web page	Sharing of documents using courseware management systems, or other applications that allow real-time document sharing
Discussion	Listservs, threaded discussions, newsgroups, e-mail	Chat rooms, real-time videoconferencing
Presentations	Multimedia or electronic presentations, case study, video tutorials, Webcasts, text-based tutorials, interactive tutorials	Real-time videoconference streaming, audio/document sharing
Evaluation	Online surveys, tests, threaded discussions, newsgroups, listservs, document sharing of assignments via e-mail	Real-time document/audio sharing, videoconference streaming

The advantages of a distance-education program are:

- Individualized pacing with active student involvement;
- Instructional assistance during and outside regular class times;
- Multiple media formats resulting in greater interactivity;
- On time assessment, feedback, and reinforcement;
- Individualized and collaborative learning;
- Optimal use of instructor's expertise;
- Information linked to student pace and performance.

Understanding the differences between traditional learning and Internet learning is essential before undertaking an online program of any kind because students who embark on a distance education program must change their thinking about how they learn. Regardless of the technology used, certain instructional functions must exist (Heinich, Molenda, Russell, & Smaldino, 1999):

- Presentation of some information to the learner such as teacher presentation or demonstration through a medium such as video or multimedia presentations, or printed texts such as handouts.
- Student–teacher interaction such as discussion, assignments, or testing.
- Student–student interaction in small groups, pairs, threaded discussions, or group projects.

IMPORTANT THEMES

There are several themes that shape online education and the future direction of learning and teaching. These themes developed by Kearsley (2000) are interrelated and overlapping but are important for the potential student.

- Collaboration: The single biggest change that the Internet brings to education is increased collaboration between students and teachers, including diverse individuals in all parts of the world. Many activities and projects involve information-sharing activities. Even when there is no specific intent to collaborate, it often happens anyway because it is so easy to interact online.
- Connectivity: These activities include discussion boards, chat rooms, e-mail, conferences, and group projects. Students and in-

structors can easily connect across time and geographic location. Another important piece of connectivity in nursing education is that students can interact directly with experts in their field of study. This is especially important in advanced nursing practice where current protocols frequently reside on the Internet. Efficient connectivity and response times are crucial for effective learning. There are three important limits to consider with respect to response times and connectivity: (1) a learner feels connected if he/she is able to retrieve information or access a page within one-tenth of a second; (2) a learner's flow of thought will be interrupted if connection takes more than 1 second; (3) a learner will stay focused on a text-based dialogue only if the interruptions are less than 10 seconds (Williams, 1998).

• Student-centered: When experienced nurses return to school for further formal education they respond well to programs that are based on adult learning principles. These principles developed by Malcolm Knowles (1980) are based on the assumption that the student is a capable decision-maker and is an active participant rather than a passive receiver in the teaching-learning process. Teachers must recognize the value of a less hierarchical learning environment and embrace the role of facilitator as their primary function. One of the most important contributions of this work is to increase awareness of the learner's rightful place at the center of the instructional process.

• Unbounded: The Internet offers online education that eliminates the walls of the classroom. It gives students access to information and people anywhere in the world. Online education removes boundaries having to do with where and when students learn, as well as who can be a learner. This is especially important for continuing education for professional nurses.

• Virtual Community: A sense of community, whether it is the community of learners defined by a particular school or continuing education program, or a physical community such as a town or city. The Internet makes it possible to define virtual communities around common interests and work-related activities. A community is only possible if a sense of presence is created (Lombard & Ditton, 1997). For example, a form of presence known as "shared space" is the degree to which students get the impression of sharing space with a virtual site on the Internet. Audio and sound are important in creating presence; therefore, the most effective online instructional communities integrate audio technology into learning (Kramer, 1995).

• Exploration: The Internet allows learners to integrate knowledge into their own behavior and belief system and to create new knowledge and insight that can only come when there is the adventure of discovery. Many online activities involve adventure or discovery learning. Problem-based learning is an example of this type of learning activity.

• Shared Knowledge: Nursing professionals and students can tap into a vast knowledge network, and they can contribute as well. Information on the Internet is immediately available to anyone in the world at any time. Sharing knowledge is the core of education, but prior to computer networks this was only accomplished in limited ways.

• Multisensory Experience: Learning theories tell us that learning is more effective when it involves multiple sensory channels such as visuals, color, movement, sound, voice, touch, and smell. For example, Edgar Dale's classic "cone of experience" theory suggests that individuals learn approximately 10% of read material, 50% of observed demonstrations and material read, and 80% of material that is interactive (Dale, 1969). Multimedia technology is available on the Internet and can provide most kinds of learning experiences except for touch and smell. Although these experiences may not be perfect, they are often much better than traditional learning activities which are primarily based on lectures.

• Authenticity: Internet education is highly authentic in nature. Students can access actual databases and experts. This gives the educational experience relevance to the learning needs of the student. The Internet provides direct access to major repositories of research information, a critical component of nursing.

WHAT TO EXPECT WITH ONLINE LEARNING

Up until now, the primary function of a teacher has been to transfer knowledge with the student in a passive role. A majority of teaching and learning is passive and most students find this style of learning very safe and comfortable. Distance education students need to be prepared for a change in this approach. When the Internet becomes the primary vehicle for learners to obtain information and skills, classes that are primarily information transfer become obsolete. Instead the student becomes an active participant in the process. The role of the instructor is to make the information meaningful, to create a positive learning environment, to integrate knowledge into the learner's own belief system, and to create new knowledge and insight that come only when three or more learners are engaged in intense discussion and exploration.

It is highly likely that soon nursing skill development will be achieved from technology in virtual nursing skills labs. Already firemen and pilots are learning skills through simulated virtual reality videos. Those teaching in online learning environments must be prepared to deliver instruction with various online learning modalities in order to meet the diverse learning styles of individuals—similar to the preparations that are adopted in the traditional classroom setting for students with various learning styles. Teachers and students must also be prepared to create a "community" of learners by encouraging discussion, participation, and presence that may require the use of more advanced technology such as audio capability.

Most individuals interested in distance education as a means to a degree, a certificate, or for continuing education, fit school into busy professional and personal lives. Successful learners are confident, motivated, persistent, and able to assume responsibility for their own learning. Family support for the decision to participate in online learning is critical, and support from the employer is also important. Some important questions to ask before engaging in online learning are: Do I have access to technology that supports distance education, such as servers that assist distance learners? Is this technology available to users around the clock? Is technology training and ongoing support available? Does the support include online mechanisms and telephone real-person options for students? How available is access to the library and student services? Is the distance program based on a philosophy and orientation to an educational process based on theory?

Be sure to provide feedback about the online learning experience. This feedback should include the following questions:

- Is this learning experience meeting my expectations?
- How is the pace of the learning? Am I able to keep up with the work required?
- What advantages have I experienced while completing this on-line learning?
- What are the disadvantages?

In conclusion, the academic quality and legitimacy of well-designed and executed distance education programs has been proved (Lewis, 2000). Do not be afraid to reach out and try a distance education course. You will be embracing a process that will prepare you for nursing practice in the 21st century.

REFERENCES

Armstrong, M. L. (2000). Distance education: Using technology to learn. In V. K. Saba & K.A. McCormick (Eds.), *Essentials of computers for nurses: Informatics for the new millennium* (3rd ed.). New York: McGraw-Hill.

Armstrong, M. L., Gossner, B. A., & Cooper, S. S. (2000). Pots, pans, and the pearls: The nursing profession's rich history with distance education for a new century of nursing. *Journal of Continuing Education in Nursing, 31,* 63–70.

Beason, C. F. (1997). Distance learning—Education to prepare nurses for practice in the 21st century. In V. Ferguson (Ed.), *Educating the 21st century nurse: Challenges and opportunities.* New York: NLN Press.

Billings, D. M., Ward, J. W., & Penton-Cooper, L. (2001). Distance learning in nursing. *Seminars in Oncology Nursing, 17,* 48–54.

Dale, E. (1969). *Audiovisual methods in teaching* (3rd ed.). New York: Dryden Press.

Ely, D. P., Foley, A., Freeman, W., & Scheel, N. (1995). Trends in educational technology, 1991. In G. J. Anglin (Ed.), *Instructional technology: Past, present and future.* Englewood, CO: Libraries Unlimited.

Garrison, J. A., Schardt, C., & Kochi, J. K. (2000). Web-based distance continuing education: A new way of thinking for students and instructors. *Bulletin of the Medical Library Association, 88,* 211–217.

Gifford, B. R. (1995, September). *Mediated learning: A new approach to asynchronous adaptive and interactive instruction and learning.* Presentation for the NLN Council of Baccalaureate and Higher Education Programs, Milwaukee, WI.

Heinich, R., Molenda, M., Russell, J. D., & Smaldino, S. E. (1999). *Instructional media and technologies for learning.* Upper Saddle River, NJ: Simon & Schuster.

Kearsley, G. (2000). *Online education: Learning and teaching in cyberspace.* Belmont, CA: Wadsworth/Thomson Learning.

Knowles, M. S. (1980). *The modern practice of adult education: From pedagogy to androgogy.* Chicago: Follett.

Kramer, G. (1995). Sound and communication in virtual reality. In F. Biocca & M. R. Levy (Eds.), *Communication in the age of virtual reality* (pp. 259–276). Hillsdale, NJ: Lawrence Erlbaum.

Lewis, J. M. (2000). Distance education foundations. In J. M. Novotny (Ed.), *Distance education in nursing.* New York: Springer Publishing Co.

Lombard, M., & Ditton, T. (1997). At the heart of it all: The concept of presence. *Journal of Computer-Mediated Communication 3*(2), [Online]. Available: *http://www.ascusc.org/jcmc/vol3/issue2/lombard.html.*

Nichols, E. F. (1997). Educational patterns in nursing. In K. K. Chitty (Ed.), *Professional nursing: Concepts and challenges*. Philadelphia: W. B. Saunders.

Novotny, J. M., & Murley, J. (1999). Designing successful learning programs. *Nursing Leadership Forum, 4*, 10–13.

Reinert, B., & Fryback, P. (1997). Distance learning and nursing education. *Journal of Nursing Education, 36*, 421–427.

Saettler, P. (1990). *The evolution of American education technology*. Englewood, CA: Libraries Unlimited, Inc.

Williams, R. (1998). Challenges to the optimal delivery of a training program via the World Wide Web. The Training Place [Online]. Available: *http://www.training-place.com/source/wbtlimit.html*

_____ Chapter **11**

Undergraduate Issues in Distance Education

Cheryl Fisher and Patricia A. Abbott

_____

U ndergraduate nursing education is becoming increasingly available as the paradigm shift in higher education moves from the traditional classroom setting to the World Wide Web. Education via the Web (distance learning) has provided the opportunity for increased accessibility to higher education because of the convenience and flexibility afforded by this methodology. With worldwide interest in this form of learning, online approaches are shaping the future of higher education.

In the international arena, distance education allows developing countries to increase the number of students who can obtain college degrees. This is not without cost to local universities who are hard-pressed to compete with often much better funded foreign institutions. "Often, students are willing to pay ten times more to have a degree from a Western institution," says Markjk van der Wende, a researcher at the Center for Higher Education Policy Studies at the Twente University of Technology in the Netherlands. "They assume it's better" (Bollag, 2001, p. 22). Although international efforts to develop competitive online programs are growing, distinct challenges exist. For example, a lack of infrastructure, a dearth of qualified distance educators, and a limited ability to monitor the quality of educational programs all pose formidable barriers for remote students, particularly in nursing.

Nationally, many universities and colleges are examining innovative methods for nursing education. Funding constraints, demands for improved efficiency, low staff-to-student ratios, and improved computer software are all combining to produce a dramatic increase in the use and movement towards the development of nursing education for delivery via the Web (Cheek, Gillham, & Mills, 1998). In addition to the explosion of available technology, pressures from the changing nursing marketplace are driving the growth in online education for undergraduate nursing education. Enrollments in colleges and schools of nursing are down nationwide. A proliferation of new career opportunities for women, who still make up more than 90 percent of the American RN workforce, has contributed to declining enrollment in nursing programs. The lingering belief that nursing is not a secure job, hospital cost cutting, and RN layoffs under the pressures of managed care, have further diminished the number of nursing students (AACN, 2000).

In reality, today's workforce situation is the exact reverse, with an increased demand for baccalaureate and graduate-prepared nurses being felt throughout the health care industry. The impact of an aging population, coupled with rapid expansion of front-line primary care and higher numbers of registered nurses (RNs) approaching retirement, has led to mounting shortages of RNs across the nation. The need to increase the number of nurses is further compounded by a federal advisory panel that has recommended that at least two-thirds of the basic nurse workforce hold baccalaureate or higher degrees in nursing by 2010. Aware of these recommendations, RNs are seeking the BSN degree in increasing numbers (AACN, 2000). Both of these challenges (the need to attract new nurses while also facilitating the movement of the RN to BSN) are exerting pressure on the current educational system. This intense need for educated nurses has fueled investigation into different ways of not only attracting students, but also in finding alternative and more flexible ways of offering nursing education.

UNDERGRADUATE NURSING EDUCATION VIA THE WEB

The demands of a dynamic health care environment and the changing profile of the student nurse have prompted universities to change or alter their traditional program offerings.

STUDENT CONSIDERATIONS IN UNDERGRADUATE NURSING EDUCATION ON THE WEB

For students, the primary advantage of completing a degree online is the access and convenience of "anytime, anywhere" education. The flexibility of distance learning for the nursing student offers a great appeal in light of busy working adult life styles and the opportunity to complete a program without having to physically drive to campus. This is particularly important for older students who are busy juggling family, school, and jobs. Many distance courses are offered "asynchronously," meaning that students can be online at any time, a flexibility greatly appreciated by busy adults. Others offer "synchronous" chat rooms or office hours, which allow students to communicate in real time with instructors or classmates. Most programs combine synchronous and asynchronous approaches. A combination of both formats can lead to enhanced learning and socialization.

Other student considerations in Web-based education include the amount of work expected and the quality of the educational experience. In a study by Leasure, Davis, and Thievon (2000) it was shown that students were concerned about the differences in the quality and quantity of learning that would take place in a Web-based undergraduate nursing research course. Students who chose not to participate in Web-based courses cited perceptions of decreased interaction with the instructor and increased busy work. A study by Viverais-Dresler and Kutschke (1992) addressed quality and student satisfaction with the clinical portion of an undergraduate distance education program. The results indicated that the degree of student satisfaction was high and was probably attributable to the investment of considerable resources in preparing clinical teachers for their role. Baier and Mueggenburg (2001) described an undergraduate clinical course in which faculty prepared students extensively for a community health practicum. Within the online course outline, students could find detailed travel directions, orientation information, names of contact people, and pictures of the agencies that would be used for their community health experience. Faculty offered several clinical sites since the number of students was limited by each agency. The success of this course was credited to careful planning, creativity, and the use of hyperlinks in the course (such as to the Centers for Disease Control), which enhanced student learning.

The quality of a Web-based nursing program is an important consideration for the student since it is desirable to attend an accredited program. Quality programs and courses are important considerations in this day and age, especially with the recent development of the "Digital Diploma Mills" which are usually unaccredited institutions on the Web. As with enrollment at a traditional school of nursing, accreditation is a critically important piece of information that a potential student must consider.

One of the cost considerations for students pursuing a nursing degree is travel associated with commuting to class and/or relocation to an area near a major university offering a degree. This problem has been somewhat mitigated with distance education, although additional costs for telecommunications are sometimes incurred. The cost of a distance education program is about equal to that of any instructional program (Lettus, 1999). However, some universities are adding a technology fee due to the changes necessary in campus infrastructure and the need for increased student support from university personnel. Other universities are eliminating a student activities fee and adding a technology fee, thereby equating the cost.

FACULTY CONSIDERATIONS OF UNDERGRADUATE EDUCATION ON THE WEB

From a faculty perspective, the adventure of distance learning is sometimes by choice and other times not. Many faculty find they develop important insights into classroom teaching through their experiences in distance education, even if the choice to participate in distance education was not elective. Faculty may discover that although assumptions and practices are challenged and new pedagogies emerge, thinking in new ways is evoked (Diekelmann & Schulte, 2000).

The application of problem-based learning (PBL) strategies to distance education offers one of those new ways of thinking. PBL is a teaching and learning method that has been successful in medical schools worldwide (Heliker, 1994). The central underpinnings of PBL involve the analysis of real-life problems or situations that need improvement while providing a framework and a stimulus for new learning. This method provides nursing students with real-world experience in the preclinical years and a safe environment in which to practice their developing professional skills (Edwards, Hugo, Cragg, & Peterson, 1999). Many nursing programs are incorporating a PBL approach because this approach is student centered, emphasizes critical thinking, and supports distance learning. As a student-centered method, it is well-suited to the needs of distance learners and is thought to enhance student motivation and provide the element of direct involvement that distance education is sometimes thought to lack.

Promoting critical thinking skills in nurses enrolled in undergraduate degree programs presents an additional challenge for nursing faculty. Many students enter the BSN program expecting faculty to lecture and fill their heads with facts to be memorized (Mastrian & McGonigle, 1999). However, the Web-based environment offers a rich medium for the development of critical thinking skills that requires students to become active participants in the learning process. When Web-based courses are well constructed using the highly interactive nature of student-centered active learning, students develop critical thinking skills and the ability to transfer and apply information to new settings. Web-based courses have provided opportunities and richer discussions not found in traditional classrooms. In fact, Web-based classroom discussions often develop into minicommunities with discussions that do not end from day to day. This ebb and flow of conversation allows students to take charge of their learning by introducing new ideas and threads of ongoing discussion thereby leading to the development of a more in-depth understanding of the topic.

CHALLENGES OF UNDERGRADUATE NURSING EDUCATION ON THE WEB

Despite the potential isolation of the Internet and e-mail communication, computer-based technology may, ironically, facilitate the important shift from teacher-orchestrated to student-centered learning (Teikmanis & Armstrong, 2001). This recent trend in education at all levels places increasing emphasis on the role of the student in the learning process and the requirement for students to take responsibility for their own learning. The implications of this added responsibility often translate to the need for students to be more self-directed in identifying their learning needs and seeking faculty feedback (Halstead & Coudret, 2000). The development of time management skills may also require retraining or the addition of a new skill base for the student. The University of Phoenix Online, for example, offers its undergraduate courses within a 5-week time frame instead of the traditional 15-week semester. Although students only take one course at a time, this may be too great a time commitment for some working adult students. The Excelsior Model, although offered with complete flexibility, still requires travel by the students to take performance exams, which may once again be difficult or inconvenient for the working adult student.

Students must master information technology in order to participate and navigate through the online course. There is an added cost of the technology and the communication medium when using distance education approaches. Since the usual support systems of the campus such as counselors, peers, and on-site faculty are no longer physically available, students must discover how to seek access to a new system of resources (Billings, 1997). The importance of peer support, tech support, and faculty support cannot be underestimated in this environment. It is important to note however that the challenges of distance education in nursing are not simply limited to students. Faculty can face significant challenges and stress as well.

From a faculty perspective, Cravener (1999) found in a review of the literature that having students at a distance increased faculty time demands when compared with classroom courses. Faculty engaged in Web-based instruction will likely find it necessary to reevaluate their own time-management skills in order to manage online classroom demands. When teaching a traditional course, faculty usually interact with students during office hours, before and after class, and during class time. Online courses allow students to communicate with faculty 24 hours a day, 7 days a week and this is exactly what they do (Hallstead & Coudret, 2000). The time consuming tasks for faculty beyond the development of the course material include counseling students, solving technological problems, ongoing support through e-mail and telephone communications, and organizing, coordinating, and analyzing data (Rose, Frisby, Hamlin, & Jones, 2000). However, it has also been noted that with experience and time, it can take less faculty time due to the change in role from sole deliverer of material to course facilitator.

One cannot assume that all nurse educators are themselves skilled in the use of computer technology. It has been suggested that the "technophobia" among nurses and students expands to those in the academic world (Kenny, 2000). New technology requires rethinking of traditional teaching dynamics, which may be perceived as threatening. The critical part of the question, "how can we engage learners via distance learning technology?" is really "how do we engage learners in more meaningful learning activities?" (Kimball, 1998). Questions such as this require that a new mind-set for teaching emerge. The most effective strategy for accomplishing this according to Kimball is to provide access to experienced distance education faculty who can serve as coaches or peer mentors.

Evaluation is another challenge facing undergraduate nursing faculty, because there is no direct observation of skills taking place in distance education courses. However, many universities have found ways around this by offering physical assessment or skill-based courses. The University of Phoenix for example, provides students with specific guidelines and criteria for performing a physical exam and requires students to have themselves videotaped for evaluation purposes. The problem with this method is that all students may not possess the necessary physical exam equipment. Other universities have students travel to an approved site with guidelines provided for evaluation. The trend is that universities are being forced to be creative in developing solutions to hands-on courses that are essential components of undergraduate nursing education.

SUCCESSFUL EXAMPLES OF UNDERGRADUATE NURSING EDUCATION ON THE WEB

An example of a completely Web-based, asynchronous, RN to BSN program can be found at the University of Maryland School of Nursing in Baltimore. Although the course work is asynchronous, the faculty offers synchronous chat time as office hours for students who want immediate feedback to short questions. The university also offers the same courses face to face and concurrently in order to accommodate different learning styles as well as different student schedules. This model provides students flexibility and options for degree completion.

California State University in Dominguez Hills was founded in 1981 as a distance-education campus. This model has evolved into a variety of BSN options for degree completion based upon student needs. This model offers teleconferencing as well as Web-based courses. Additionally, students can take course work on campus or on a weekend schedule. This BSN program credits its success to meeting the needs of RN adult learners whose time, life styles, or work schedules might make it impossible to complete a traditional course of study in residence at a college campus. Flexibility is credited as key to success in addition to options for degree completion.

Although many Web-based, asynchronous RN to BSN programs are now available throughout the country, the University of Phoenix Online offers a unique model for its undergraduate students. This program offers courses in a 5-week framework in which students take one course at a time. The students are required to participate in the online classroom five out of seven days of the week in classes restricted to 15 students. This model forces the students to work so closely and intensely that a sense of community develops almost automatically within the first week of class.

Excelsior College has been in existence since 1971. Although it is a distance-learning program, it would be considered Web-supported. This program model is self-paced for students with no semesters or courses. The philosophy is "what you know, not how you learned." This assessment-based model provides study guides and study materials that prepare students for either a written or a performance-based exam. Once the students have completed the required preparation, they have up to 1 year to take the course exam in order to receive course credit. The student support services are Web-based, and an electronic peer network is offered which enables students the opportunity to find a "study buddy." The success of this accredited program is based on its reputation and flexibility.

DISTANCE LEARNING NURSING PROGRAM RESOURCES

Currently, the Web-based distance learning programs are primarily for degree completion or RN to BSN programs. The programs mentioned in this chapter offer a variety of courses from fully Web based to self-instruction using study guide materials. The models currently available can be categorized into fully Web based or Web supported. Recently, several organizations have developed directories of online education (Billings, Ward, & Penton-Cooper, 2001). These directories provide databased information that allows students to "shop" or identify courses or programs that are appropriate for individual needs. Some examples include *Peterson's Distance Learning* (*www.lifelonglearning.com*), the World Lecture Hall (*www.utexas.edu/world/lecture*), and *Barron's Distance Learning Guide* (available for sale online, but content is available only in written format).

Although traditional semester scheduling seems to be the predominant model with courses being offered within a 15-week time frame, it has been speculated that in the future the traditional semester walls may be a thing of the past. As distance programs strive to outdo each other in terms of offering flexibility to meet student needs, the trend in course offerings may migrate towards student determination of course start and finish times and a purely asynchronous format.

As more distance nursing programs emerge (currently over 200 according to Petersons.com distance learning database) in some varying form, the trend appears to be that all universities desire to have this option available to offer potential students. The Indiana College Network stated that they have several calls a week from prospective students both in and out of state inquiring about the availability of their distance learning programs. Although this method of learning may never replace the traditional classroom, it does offer students the opportunity to further their higher education in ways not available in the past. As more research is conducted on ways to improve Web-based distance learning, the availability and quality of nursing education can be expected to broaden and improve.

CONCLUSIONS

When teaching at a distance, there are changes in how faculty manage their time, calculate workload, explain productivity, and produce evidence of teaching for promotion and merit raise decisions (Billings, 1997). Student roles also change, since students need to be more responsible for their learning and need to learn how to use technology as a means of supporting their learning. The challenge for educators, according to Kenny (2000), is to incorporate the technology into teaching and use it to assist and enhance the ability to prepare nursing students to meet the demands of professional nursing practice. As distance learning continues to expand offerings to students across state lines and continents, the benefits of flexibility, availability, and choice will encourage lifelong learning and allow students to view technology as the means to further education.

WEB SITE RECAP

Peterson's Distance Learning
http://www.lifelonglearning.com

World Lecture Hall
http://www.utexas.edu/world/lecture

REFERENCES

AACN (2000). Strategies to reverse the new nursing shortage. [Online]. Available: *http://www.aacn.nche.edu/Media/Backgrounders/nursfact.htm.*

Baier, M., & Mueggenburg, K. (2001). Using the Internet for clinical instruction. *Nurse Educator, 26*, 3.

Billings, D. (1997). Issues in teaching and learning at a distance: Changing role. *Computers in Nursing, 15*(2), 69–70.

Billings, D., Ward, J., & Penton-Cooper, L. (2001). Distance learning in nursing. *Seminars in Oncology Nursing, 17*(1), 48–54.

Bollag, B. (2001). Developing countries turn to distance education. *Chronicle of Higher Education.* [Online]. Available: http://chronicle.com.

Cheek, J., Gillham, D., & Mills, P. (1998). Use with care: Possibilities and constraints offered by computers in nursing clinical education. *International Journal of Medical Information, 50*(1–3), 111–115.

Cravener, P. (1999). Faculty experiences with providing online courses: Thorns among the roses. *Computers in Nursing, 17*(1), 42–47.

Diekelmann, N., & Schulte, H. D. (2000). Technology-based distance education and the absence of physical presence. *Journal of Nursing Education, 39*(2), 51–52.

Edwards, N., Hugo, K., Cragg, B., & Peterson, J. (1999). The integration of problem-based learning strategies in distance education. *Nurse Educator, 24*(1), 36–41.

Halstead, J., & Coudret, N. (2000). Implementing Web-based instruction in a school of nursing: Implications for faculty and students. *Journal of Professional Nursing, 16*, 273–281.

Heliker, D. (1994). Meeting the challenge of the curriculum revolution: Problem-based learning in nursing education. *Journal of Nursing Education, 33*(1), 45–47.

Kenny, A. (2000). Untangling the Web: Barriers and benefits for nurse education; an Australian perspective. *Nurse Education Today, 20*, 381–388.

Kimball, L. (1998). Managing distance learning—new challenges for faculty. In R. Hazeim, S. Hailes, & S. Wilbur (Eds.), *The digital university: Reinventing the academy* (pp. 25–37). London: Springer.

Leasure, R., Davis, L., & Thievon, S. (2000). Comparison of student outcomes and preference in a traditional vs. World Wide Web based baccalaureate nursing research course. *Journal of Nursing Education, 39*, 149–154.

Lettus, M. (1999) Distance education—is it right for you? *Imprint, 46*(2), 39–41.

Mastrian, K., & McGonigle, D. (1999). Using technology-based assignments to promote critical thinking. *Nurse Educator, 24*(1), 45–47.

Rose, M., Frisby, A., Hamlin, M., & Jones, S. (2000). Evaluation of the effectiveness of a Web-based graduate epidemiology course. *Computers in Nursing, 18*, 162–167.

Teikmanis, M., & Armstrong, J. (2001). Teaching pathophysiology to diverse students using an online discussion board. *Computers in Nursing, 19*, 75–81.

Viverais-Dresler, G., & Kutschke, M. (1992). RN students' satisfaction with clinical teaching in a distance education program. *Journal of Continuing Education in Nursing, 23*, 224–230.

Chapter **12**

Graduate Issues in Distance Education

Maureen Gerrity, Janice L. Gibson, and Patricia A. Abbott

N urses today are working in a rapidly changing environment in which knowledge becomes quickly outdated. Thus, they must learn how to use the available technology proficiently to access resources on the Internet. Furthermore, students of higher education need learning experiences that will help them develop effective critical thinking skills, as well as the ability to obtain current information and knowledge on an ongoing basis.

It is becoming clear that the use of electronic communications technologies will become an integral part of the educational landscape. The World Wide Web provides a rich resource of health-related information that can be used to promote and enhance student learning. Once thought of primarily as a means to deliver distance education, Web-enhanced instruction is becoming increasingly mainstream in higher education (Halstead & Coudret, 2000). Students enrolled in Web-based courses experience a more independent, self-directed approach to learning that is consistent with the graduate education goal of lifelong professional learning. Increased knowledge of the Internet and skills gained by students enrolled in Web-enhanced courses are essential learning outcomes for advanced practice nurses.

The primary reason for nursing schools to offer Web-based programs however, is the need for distance education. This need has arisen because nurses who are returning for additional degrees are employed and have family responsibilities (Billings, 2000). In addition, distance education is essential to transcend geographic barriers limiting work-

141

force development in rural areas or where advanced practice nurses are in short supply.

In this chapter, we discuss application of the Internet to graduate education, various models for providing graduate education using Internet resources, as well as benefits, limitations, needed resources, and practical considerations for using the Internet. Issues related to cost and future research are also discussed.

APPLICATIONS OF THE INTERNET TO GRADUATE EDUCATION

Graduate students today, especially returning, older students, are demanding access to courses that will allow them to remain in the workforce and meet family responsibilities while pursuing advanced education. Many schools of nursing address these demands by offering distance education using video teleconferencing via satellite. The disadvantage of this delivery system is that it requires students to travel to a designated location at a specific time for their weekly classes. Work schedules that include shift rotations, twelve-hour shifts, on-call periods, and mandatory overtime make it difficult for nurses to commit to regular classroom attendance at a specified time. Asynchronous instruction, on the other hand, can enable students at remote sites to complete an entire program of study in their own home, at their own pace, and at any time or day they choose.

When considering the educational needs of graduate students, one must give particular attention to the specific needs of the adult learner. Norman (1997) emphasized the need to consider a variety of variables when designing an online course, including the depth and complexity of the material, the autonomy and motivation of the learner, the emphasis on discovery and exploration, and the importance of learning criteria.

An important advantage of distance learning via the Web is that it allows for a "constructivist" approach to learning. This approach encourages a change in focus from teacher-dominated instruction to student-centered learning (Norman, 1997). Graduate students enter the classroom with their own experiences and a cognitive structure based on those experiences. The learner will reformulate his or her existing structures only if new information or experiences are connected to knowledge already in memory. Memorized facts or information that has not been connected with the learner's prior experiences will be quickly forgotten. As the learner integrates previously acquired experiences and knowledge with the current learning situation, new constructs are formed (Vuono, 1998). The constructivist approach can be fostered in a Web-based course through online communications among class participants.

Asynchronous communications using a software conferencing system can become the center of learning if a problem-based learning approach is used. Case studies can be presented through an online seminar where students can work in virtual groups or individually to process content and develop solutions to the identified problems. This approach requires an active learning style for students using constructivist principles, yet the communications may remain asynchronous, permitting nurses with even the most challenging work schedules to remain in school.

It is especially important for advanced practice nurses to be able to obtain the latest health care information. Medical, nursing, and other health related, online journals and databases now provide immediate access to research findings and treatment protocols. In addition, patients are using the Internet to seek health care information, frequently presenting this information to their health care providers. Increasingly, advanced practice nurses will be called upon to deliver health services via various forms of technology such as telehealth. Thus, they must have the computer skills necessary to locate Internet resources (Halstead & Coudret, 2000).

MODELS FOR GRADUATE EDUCATION USING INTERNET RESOURCES

Geibert (2000) views Web-enhanced instruction as an effective adjunct to videoconferencing to enhance collaborative opportunities. In this model, Web technology is used to create learning communities and support learner-centered strategies for students in on-campus courses. The advantage to this approach is the multiplicity of communication methods employed to enable students to communicate in a variety of ways. An additional advantage of using multiple systems is that students were able to continue their academic pursuits even if one of the systems experienced technical failure.

According to Geibert (2000), faculty feedback after the first semester indicated that the tools provided by Web-enhanced instruction were instrumental in helping students submit collaborative work that often far exceeded faculty expectations. Geibert's data support the conclusion that the integration of Web-enhanced instruction to support collaboration in the graduate nursing program met or exceeded desired outcomes.

Faculty at the Ball State University School of Nursing have also decided on a mix of classroom and Web delivery of course content. Carlton, Ryan, and Siktberg (1998) report that their mix will be course dependent, but the objective is to deliver approximately two-thirds of the course electronically and one-third in the classroom. Classroom time provides the opportunity for orientation to the course, presentations by students, and clinical labs. According to these authors, faculty highly value classroom time, because they believe that "personal contact with graduate students is important, both between faculty and students and among students" (Carlton, Ryan, & Siktberg, 1998, p. 49).

Iwasiw and colleagues (2000) described a collaborative project designed to provide an international educational experience for graduate students studying nursing administration using distance-learning technologies. This Web-enhanced project, known as the "Canada-Norway Nursing Connection," employed video teleconferencing to connect in both countries. Computer conferencing was used for students to engage in case study discussion. These authors used tenets of the social constructivist paradigm to design the project. The conceptual basis for this educational experience stemmed from the belief that students' collaborative efforts of collecting and sharing information and experiences would be transformed into knowledge that maintained personal meaning and relevance.

Albrektson (1995) advocates the use of asynchronous online discussion for a graduate-level seminar course. It was noted that students assumed ownership of the online discussions and participated in more than the minimum as required by the course. These learners became more self-directed in pursuing educational outcomes, even citing literature to support their statements. Teikmanis and Armstrong (2001) also described a successful implementation of an online discussion group. This was done to overcome the barriers to class participation for a pathophysiology course that was conducted in large lecture fashion.

A unique example of a Web-enhanced course is described by authors from Johns Hopkins University in Baltimore and San Diego State University (Nolan, Morrison, Riegel, & Thomason, 1999). This application arose when a student who had completed all of the requirements for her graduate degree except for the capstone course, moved to California. Because this course was meant to integrate the content of the entire program, it could not easily be substituted with a course from another university. Furthermore, it did not readily lend itself to traditional distance-educational strategies because of the clinical component. The solution involved collaboration between faculty from both schools using e-mail communication to plan and teach the course. The Johns Hopkins faculty member was kept apprised of the student's clinical experiences by way of e-mail; however, the hope of generating communication between the other students in the class was never realized. The lack of structured, online communications among all students resulted in a missed opportunity for the California student to learn from fellow classmates' clinical experiences.

In a similar sequence of events during the fall 2000 and spring 2001 semesters at the University of Maryland School of Nursing, desktop video was used to link distant students and their seminar participants during their capstone course in the Nursing Informatics graduate program. Desktop video, involving a video card and a small camera on top of the computers, was used at both the student sites and the classroom site. Microsoft's NetMeeting was the format used, which permitted two-way transmission of both audio and video. Although the transmission quality and the view range of the camera were limited, this approach provided the most cost-effective means for providing videoconferencing. This course utilized other Web-enhanced strategies to link students in all locations, including a class Web page, e-mail, and a course listserv.

Mills (2000) described a Web-based program conducted at the St. Louis University School of Nursing. The school was awarded a program extension grant to expand its existing family nurse practitioner program by offering the program online. WebCT (Universal Learning Technology, Inc., Andover, MA) was selected as the course building software. The software contains a set of designer tools to produce the layout of the course, and to organize and sequence classes and presentations. A program template was developed to produce each course with a similar appearance and function, thereby minimizing the time required for students to orient themselves (Mills, 2000). Course pages were designed using hypertext mark-up language (HTML). Selected documents were converted to portable document format (PDF) files and viewed by students using free Acrobat Reader software. Hypertext links appropriate to specific class content were integrated for these courses, and audiovisual elements were incorporated into the format, thus maximizing the Web's multimedia capacity.

ADVANTAGES OF USING THE INTERNET IN GRADUATE EDUCATION

The most frequently noted advantage of using the Internet in graduate education is the ability to transcend time and space barriers. This is of great benefit to nurses since it can accommodate the lifestyles and work schedules of those who desire formal learning opportunities. Graduate students, in particular, appreciate the ability to study on an independent schedule and welcome the opportunity to be self-directed (Dawes, 1998). In addition, it provides wider access to academic institutions and maximizes access to qualified instructors.

Graduate-level group project work is greatly facilitated by Internet access since communication can occur asynchronously. Project files can be quickly and easily shared with group members as e-mail attachments. Dede (1996) believes enhanced team performance results as learners work and communicate collaboratively in an online environment. Tools that may be used to communicate ideas also provide structure for group dialogue and maintain a record of the rationale used by the group to make choices. Computer-supported, collaborative methodologies are particularly helpful for individual work on group projects since it allows the continuation of work from the student's home.

Halstead and Coudret (2000) found that students valued the self-paced, independent learning experience afforded by Web-enhanced education. Harasim, Hiltz, Teles, and Turoff (1996, in Geibert, 2000) found that learning became more individualized when computer-mediated communication was used. This independence can be a double-edged sword, however, as the lack of structure requires more self-discipline on the part of the student. Some students report that they are not comfortable with the lack of classroom structure (Dawes, 1998).

Carlton, Ryan, and Siktberg (1998) highlighted the benefits of using an online bulletin board to enhance group discussion of a topic using a case study format. They found that critical thinking skills were enhanced because case studies required synthesis, analysis, and evaluation for application to the scenarios. In addition, this medium provides each student the opportunity to review case studies and respond to others on a given topic. In the classroom setting this does not always occur since shy students may not participate in the discussion, while others tend to dominate. Halstead and Coudret (2000) found that students are more likely to participate in computer-mediated discussion than they are in a classroom setting. Thiele, Allen, and Stuckey (1999) reported that faculty found students were more likely to ask questions or disagree with the instructor when engaged in online dialogue.

Iwasiw and colleagues (2000) emphasized the importance of expanding the instruction of graduate students in nursing administration to include perspectives on nursing leadership and administration across borders and cultures. Using the powerful alternatives offered by distance technologies, the Canada-Norway Nursing Connection project provided an international learning experience without the need for learner relocation. The high costs associated with travel, sometimes prohibitive, were avoided while discussions of the global forces influencing the profession were made possible through the use of the Internet and videoconferencing.

Halstead and Coudret (2000) identified additional student-perceived benefits in a survey following an online course. Students valued the increased time flexibility as well as decreased travel time. Further, they cited improved computer skills, increased access to information, and self-paced, independent learning.

In the same study, Halstead and Coudret identified faculty-perceived advantages following Web-based instruction. Although faculty found that an online course resulted in increased time demands for teaching the course, it offered the advantage of having increased time flexibility. In addition, they cited increased access to course-related, cutting-edge information, increased frequency of communication with individual students, and increased frequency and depth of student contributions to class discussion. In Dawes's research (1998), faculty who had taught distance education courses noted as benefits increased interest in and reflection about their own pedagogical practices, opportunities to reach new students, and state and national recognition. Finally, promotion, tenure, and merit recognition were cited by faculty as advantages for teaching online courses.

DISADVANTAGES OF USING THE INTERNET IN GRADUATE EDUCATION

Despite the many advantages of using the Internet in graduate education, this venture should be entered into with full comprehension of the disadvantages and a plan to resolve potential problems. As Link and Scholtz (2000) pointed out, although faculty members are aware of consumer demand for asynchronous programs and the advantages they offer to both students and the university, they may be less than enthusiastic about this means of instruction. Although the seminal literature regarding computer anxiety was produced in the late 1980s and early 1990s, it is still an issue with both faculty and students, as evidenced by current literature, conference proceedings, and anecdotal reports from educators and trainers (Geibert, 2000).

Halstead and Coudret (2000) found that although faculty were comfortable using e-mail, few were actually using the Internet for teaching. Clearly, however, faculty must be skilled in the use of the tools available to create these courses and comfortable operating the hardware required to run them. Yucha and Princen (2000) highlight the computer literacy issue for students as well, reminding us that many graduate students in nursing finished high school and received their BSN degrees before computer literacy was required and before Web-based instruction was available.

Halstead and Coudret (2000) point out that faculty who have considerable experience with traditional classroom teaching, and who gain professional satisfaction through their personal classroom interactions with students, may find it particularly difficult to engage in Web-based instruction. Relying on computer-mediated communication for instructional purposes is a new experience for most faculty and students, and may initially appear to be impersonal or result in a lack of participation in the course. Furthermore, engaging in Web-based instruction requires faculty to completely reconceptualize their role.

Several authors discuss the lack of personal interaction as a disadvantage of Web-based instruction as perceived by students (Dawes, 1998; Halstead & Coudret, 2000). Students frequently cite decreased peer interaction, and feelings of isolation and alienation as disadvantages. In addition, they may experience a sense of isolation and separation from the institution itself. These feelings are the reason for the high attrition rates for this type of instruction, according to Link and Scholtz (2000).

The exclusive use of written communications for online discussions presents significant challenges for both faculty and students where clarity of communications is concerned. Without voice intonation and body language to help them, students with poor written communication skills may find the task too challenging for their participation (Teikmanis & Armstrong, 2001). This may be particularly difficult for individuals for whom English is a second language. Langford and Harden (1999) remind us that typed messages must be accurately and carefully stated. The choice of words must be expressive, explicit, and unambiguous. Electronic communications are not as tolerant of the use of slang and grammatical inaccuracies as face-to-face interactions are.

Chat rooms, which allow for the use of synchronous communications, present another set of problems. Because these discussions are typed messages and are conducted in real-time, they frequently result in several conversations going on at once. This occurs, when several individuals are responding at the same time to comments made by different participants.

Issues related to technology present a major disadvantage to relying on the Internet for a course. Given the unpredictability of the Internet and computers in general, it can be guaranteed that technical problems will develop during a course using online resources. Technology difficulties can be highly frustrating for both students and faculty and can greatly undermine the success of using Internet resources for graduate education.

PRACTICAL CONSIDERATIONS

Students' feelings of alienation, lack of connectedness, and isolation from faculty and other students are a significant drawback to the use of online courses. Faculty must be in touch with students on a regular basis and encourage interaction among the students to improve the odds that students will complete the course (Link & Scholtz, 2000). Halstead and Coudret (2000) add that students feel more individually connected to the faculty and the course when they receive timely responses to their questions.

Halstead and Coudret (2000) suggest a number of electronic methods to promote communication, such as the establishment of weekly "office hours" when they will be available to answer student questions promptly via e-mail or by phone. Posting answers to commonly asked questions in a public format such as a listserv allows other students to read and benefit from the answers. Halstead and Coudret also suggests that faculty require students to identify personal learning goals for the course and send them by e-mail during the first week. This may help break the ice and give faculty information that they can use to begin building a relationship with individual students.

By creating an online learning community for students, educators can help counter students' feelings of isolation (Palloff & Pratt, 1999). Generating a sense of excitement about learning together, an online learning community supports and encourages knowledge acquisition, and supports the intellectual as well as personal growth and development of its members. "The total outcome of knowledge acquired and shared is far greater than what would be generated through independent, individual engagement with the material" (Palloff & Pratt, 1999, p. 163).

Halstead and Coudret (2000) suggest that situations involving failed technology can best be handled by expecting that difficulties will occur and actively developing strategies for managing them. These authors suggest developing alternate learning activities for those instances when technical problems arise. It is also suggested that faculty assign less technically challenging activities for the first couple of weeks of the course, placing more demanding assignments later in the course. "Students can become overwhelmed quickly as they try to cope with technical difficulties at the same time they are trying to learn large amounts of new material" (Halstead & Coudret, 2000, p. 278). Arranging for availability of campus technical support will enable both students and faculty to devote their attention to course content rather than technology issues.

Both faculty and students engaged in Web-based instruction will likely find it necessary to reevaluate and refine their time management skills. When teaching a traditional course, faculty ordinarily establishes office hours around scheduled class meetings. However, an online course allows students to communicate with faculty 24 hours a day, seven days week. Faculty can no longer easily compartmentalize student contact within an established time frame and can find themselves inundated with e-mail messages and online discussions (Halstead & Coudret, 2000). These authors suggest that the instructor develop individual e-mail folders for each student in the course, allowing them to easily file and retrieve each student's work at their convenience.

Halstead and Coudret (2000) also offer suggestions for managing online discussions. Since it is not reasonable for faculty to provide responses to all comments posed by students, their comments should be limited to those that "move the discussion to the next level of analysis, introduce information that students may be overlooking, provide constructive feedback, and help summarize key discussion points" (p. 277).

Since enrolling in a Web course is a new experience, most students will find that they must learn new time management habits in order to keep up with course work. Online courses require that students be more self-directed and actively seek faculty feedback, since the structure of the classroom does not exist (Dawes, 1998).

RESOURCES NEEDED TO USE THE INTERNET IN GRADUATE NURSING EDUCATION

Whether instituting a Web-based or Web-enhanced course, a number of resources are necessary to help ensure a successful outcome. These include state-of-the-art hardware and software, time, and adequate technical assistance. While most online courseware contains many of the tools to conduct a Web-based course, the Internet can provide applications for enhancing a traditional classroom or videoconferencing course. Computer conferencing software is useful for synchronous, open discussion of course content. For discussion of particular topics of interest, individual conference rooms can be set up and devoted to selected course content.

Bulletin boards can be utilized for asynchronous, threaded discussions. For many students this is a novel experience and may initially need some encouragement to participate. Specific assignments can be structured to include the online discussion format by asking students, for example, to share their own insights around a specific topic. Halstead and Coudret (2000) found that specific assignments frequently generated interesting and meaningful dialogue among students as they compared their experiences. A course home page can be used that includes links to some of the rich resources available on the Web. An annotated hyperlink list with links to online databases and library catalogs might also be included.

Access to an e-mail system by all students and faculty is a useful tool for establishing private communications. It can be used by faculty for such things as the delivery of course materials, giving individual student feedback, and for sending assignment reminders. Students can use e-mail for sending assignments to faculty and for communications with fellow group members concerning project work. A course listserv provides all members of the class and faculty with a means for sending information to, or requesting information from, the entire class at once by way of e-mail. Caution must be used, however, when adding attachments to e-mail because of the risk of viruses and worms.

According to Link and Scholtz (2000), use of the Web for teaching has created a whole new set of workload considerations that must be understood and addressed. Time must be invested by faculty to learn to use the technology tools necessary for Internet learning applications. It also takes time to read and evaluate students' online discussions, post questions, and participate in threaded discussions (Teikmanis & Armstrong, 2001).

An orientation to course software and tools is recommended for both faculty and students. Geibert (2000) suggests that as part of the orientation, each student enrolled in an online course should receive a letter identifying skills and resources necessary to be successful in the course. Suggested requirements include access to a computer with an Internet connection, a personal e-mail address, completion of a basic computer course, the ability to use a word processing program, and experience using a Web browser. Since bandwidth issues can contribute to student frustration during an online course, students should be encouraged to avoid this obstacle by utilizing DSL or cable lines for their Internet access. Online tutorials to introduce students to basic computer skills necessary for an online course might include an introduction to the course software, Internet basics, use of e-mail, Web publishing, and online chat.

Halstead and Coudret (2000) believe that students and faculty are justified in their concern that dealing with technology-related issues will overshadow course content and negatively affect faculty effectiveness and student learning. Parker (1997) found that one of the obstacles to increased use of technology by faculty was the lack of on-site access to computer experts. Access to university technical support personnel can also help reduce student time spent dealing with technical issues and allow more time and energy to be focused on course content. In addition to access to technical support, Halstead and Coudret (2000) found it beneficial to employ an HTML coding expert. They point out that because not all institutions have the resources to keep an expert on staff, course development and editing software can provide templates to aid in course design and management, thus eliminating the need for faculty to have advanced knowledge of HTML.

COST ISSUES

Administrators in institutions of higher education who introduce online courses and programs with the belief that they are low-cost, high-revenue ventures are mistaken, according to Link and Scholtz (2000). Offering Web-based courses involves significant costs for faculty, technical experts, and maintenance of the sophisticated technologic infrastructure.

Halstead and Coudret (2000) believe that there is a misconception that the use of Web-based course delivery will allow institutions to increase student enrollment, thereby increasing tuition revenues. On the contrary, they have found that Web-based courses increase the amount of faculty time spent in course preparation and delivery, and thus, in some cases, may actually require a reduction in the number of students who may enroll in a given course. This is necessary to maintain the desired quality of instruction and level of student satisfaction. The authors report further that enrollment in their Web-based courses typically ranges from 25 to 40 students, the same as in their traditional, classroom-based courses. Zhang (1998) agrees that class size should be kept relatively low to remain manageable for the instructor. She believes the maximum ratio of students to faculty should be 15:1, with 8:1 being optimal.

Billings (1996a) disagrees with the assessment that online courses do not increase revenues, saying that although there is an initial investment in course development, ongoing use and delivery of the instructional materials is relatively inexpensive. Furthermore, Billings believes that offering online courses serves as a powerful vehicle for recruitment and retention for schools of nursing, thereby increasing tuition revenues. She adds that recruitment advantages are gained by remote students' access to experts, and salary savings are achieved since faculty are not employed in multiple sites. Carlton, Ryan, and Siktberg (1998) agree that Web-based courses can help sustain the viability of universities in the face of limited state and federal funding resources.

FUTURE DIRECTIONS

The next generation of nursing students will most likely receive much of their high-school and college education via the Internet. Being prepared for this generation as they enter graduate school will require that time and resources be directed toward developing faculty and the technical infrastructure to support the demand for sophisticated learning environments. Administrators should begin now to ensure that opportunities exist for faculty to discuss newly emerging teaching and learning technologies and strategies (Langford & Harden, 1999).

Gaining an understanding of nursing and health care issues in an international context will become increasingly important in the future as the global economy continues to evolve. Advanced practice nurses will require a global perspective in order to become the leaders and problem-solvers of the future.

Videoconferencing and Internet technologies currently provide the technical means for international graduate-level nursing education. Advanced voice recognition systems will likely replace keyboards in the future, allowing for improved, real-time, online discussions, and the ability to transcend language barriers.

Virtual reality applications are now becoming available for the teaching of certain tasks and procedures through Web-based courses (Langford & Hardin, 1999). Combined with the advanced technology of the Internet, they will allow more and more nursing education to take place in remote locations, far away from faculty role models. Salmon (1999) cautions that nursing curricula must identify critical clinical and nonclinical skills that must remain separate from technology so as not to displace the core value of caring that is the cornerstone of nursing.

FUTURE RESEARCH

Clearly there is disagreement in the literature about the ideal class size for an online course, as well as the cost-effectiveness of this type of delivery, making online education a fruitful area for future nursing research. Teikmanis and Armstrong (2001) agree that nurses should study class size to determine what is indeed manageable, particularly for the effective use of electronic discussions. Furthermore, the authors would like to know whether participation in these discussions increases student learning in a measurable way. Finally, Billings (1996b) questions whether electronic communications in the classroom promotes the type of communication skills that advanced practice nurses need.

SUMMARY

Distance learning technologies offer powerful and creative alternatives to traditional classroom graduate nursing education. These advanced mechanisms for learning transcend geographic boundaries, time and schedule limitations, and many other access issues by using the Internet and the Web. Sharing of information and experiences, and knowledge transfer are enhanced, and can be offered either in real time or via an asynchronous communications environment. Design and implementation approaches to distance learning may vary, offering some degree of customization depending on needs. While this technology broadens the educational landscape and offers an enriched, global perspective on the forces affecting the nursing profession, both student and faculty requirements for online course participation must be identified and addressed prior to jumping on the virtual university bandwagon.

REFERENCES

Albrektson, J. R. (1995). Mentored online seminar: A model for graduate-level distance education. *T. H. E. Journal*, 102–105.

Billings, D. (1996a). Connecting points: Distance education in nursing. *Computers in Nursing, 14*, 211–212, 217.

Billings, D. (1996b). Connecting points: Distance education in nursing—adapting courses for distance education. *Computers in Nursing, 14*, 262–263, 266.

Billings, D. (2000). A framework for assessing outcomes and practices in Web-based courses in nursing. *Journal of Nursing Education, 39*(2), 60–67.

Carlton, K., Ryan, M., & Siktberg, L. (1998). Designing courses for the Internet. *Nurse Educator, 23*(3), 45–50.

Dawes, B. S. G. (1998). Can distance learning provide a twenty-first century hallmark? *Association for PeriOperative Registered Nurses Journal, 68*, 170–174.

Dede, C. (1996). Emerging technologies in distance education for business. *Journal of Education for Business, 71*, 197–204.

Geibert, R. C. (2000). Integrating Web-based instruction into a graduate nursing program taught via videoconferencing—challenges and solutions. *Computers in Nursing, 18*, 26–34.

Halstead, J., & Coudret, N. (2000). Implementing Web-based instruction in a school of nursing: Implications for the faculty and students. *Journal of Professional Nursing, 16*, 273–281.

Iwasiw, C., Andrusyszyn, M. A., Moen, A., Ostbye, T., Davie, L., Stovring, T., & Buckland-Foster, I. (2000). Graduate education in nursing leadership through distance technologies: The Canada-Norway nursing connection. *Journal of Nursing Education, 39*(2), 81–86.

Langford, D., & Hardin, S. (1999). Distance learning: Issues emerging as the paradigm shifts. *Nursing Science Quarterly, 12*, 191–196.

Link, D., & Scholtz, S. (2000). Educational technology and the faculty role: What you don't know can hurt you. *Nurse Educator, 25*, 274–276.

Mills, A. (2000). Creating Web-based, multimedia, and interactive courses for distance learning. *Computers in Nursing, 18*, 125–131.

Nolan, M., Morrison, J., Riegel, B., & Thomason, T. (1999). Spotlight on: Support of an off-site student through collaboration and e-mail. *Nurse Educator, 24*, 8–10.

Norman, K. L. (1997). Teaching in the switched on classroom: An introduction to electronic education and hypercourseware. [Online]. Available: *http://www.lap.umd.edu/SOC/sochome.html.*

Palloff, R. M., & Pratt, K. (1999). *Building learning communities in cyberspace.* San Francisco: Jossey-Bass.

Parker, D. (1997). Increasing faculty use of technology in teaching and teacher education. *Journal of Technology and Teacher Education, 5*(2/3), 105–115.

Salmon, M. (1999). Thoughts on nursing: Where it has been and where it is going. *Nursing and Healthcare Perspectives, 20*, 20–25.

Teikmanis, M., & Armstrong, J. (2001). Teaching pathophysiology to diverse students using an online discussion board. *Computers in Nursing, 19*, 75–82.

Thiele, J. E., Allen, C., & Stuckey, M. (1999). Effects of Web-based instruction on learning behaviors of undergraduate and graduate students. *Nursing and Health Care Perspectives, 20*, 199–203.

Vuono, M. M. (1998). Distance learning in graduate nursing. [Online]. Available: *http://parsons.umaryland.edu/journal/v2n1/vuono/html.*

Yucha, C., & Princen, M. A. (2000). Insights learned from teaching pathophysiology on the World Wide Web. *Journal of Nursing Education, 39*(2), 68–72.

Zhang, P. (1998). A case study on technology use in distance learning. *Journal of Research on Computing in Education, 30*, 398–415.

Chapter 13

Issues for Advanced Practice Students

Jane Koeckeritz

The role of the advanced practice nurse has developed and evolved over an extended period of time. Each of the four roles, nurse anesthetist, certified nurse midwife, clinical nurse specialist, and nurse practitioner has its own unique history. The last decade of the 20th century brought major growth in all fields of advanced practice nursing, however. As these roles took shape and a niche for each was created, the term advanced practice nurse gained widespread acceptance. The American Nurses Association (ANA) officially defined the role of advanced practice nurse in 1992. The ANA definition of advanced clinical nursing practice reads:

> Nurses in advanced clinical practice have a graduate degree in nursing. They conduct comprehensive health assessments, demonstrate a high level of autonomy, and possess expert skills in the diagnosis and treatment of complex responses of individuals, families, and communities to actual or potential health problems. They formulate clinical decisions to manage acute and chronic illness and promote wellness. Nurses in advanced practice integrate education, research, management, leadership, and consultation into their clinical roles and function in collegial relationships with nursing peers, physicians, professionals, and others who influence the health environment. (Berger et al., 1996, p. 250)

This definition informs advanced practice nurse educators as to the knowledge, skills, and abilities (KSA) expected of program graduates as they begin their clinical practice. Accomplishing the task of educating students for these roles is challenging. As the students graduate, they move into practices that are complex and constantly changing. In this changing health care environment, health care providers can never make the assumption that they have completed their education. The focus of graduate education cannot be simply on content but must also include the development of attitudes and skills that ensure lifelong learning. The role of the Internet in clinical practice and as a tool for lifelong learning is an essential part of the education of advanced practice nurses. Providing students with the KSA to maximize Web resources and make the Internet an important part of their everyday practice is the responsibility of advanced practice nurse educators.

HISTORICAL PERSPECTIVE

The major growth of the Internet as a tool to support nursing education, research, and clinical practice did not occur until the 1990s. Nursing literature prior to the past decade had little information about the Internet since up to that point it was of limited value to nursing. This relatively recent use of the Internet and the Web in health care has been explosive and has resulted in telemedicine and telehealth moving from the periphery to center stage in a very short time (Bauer & Ringel, 1999).

Current faculty in schools of nursing throughout the country were well established in their careers and faculty positions before the Internet became a part of everyday life. Degree programs completed by the majority of today's advanced practice faculty did not include technology as a necessary skill for graduation. This has resulted in a lag in the infusion of these technologies into many advanced practice curricula. This trend is changing as information technology skills are being recognized as critical to best practice.

APPLICATION OF THE INTERNET IN APN EDUCATION

Advanced practice nurses work in a variety of roles including clinician, educator, researcher, manager, and consultant. It is common for advanced practice nurses to be expected to function in a variety of these roles within one employment setting. Given the magnitude of knowledge required for competent practice in these diverse roles, APN educators must provide a framework in which students learn to utilize resources for practice, education, research, and administration. The

Internet is replete with resources supporting the many functions of the advanced practice nurse.

Clinician

The most obvious role of the advanced practice nurse is that of care provider. Superb skills in assessment, diagnostic reasoning, planning, referral, and evaluation are required. Teaching these skills necessitates an interactive educational process that provides role models and encourages participation and questioning. It is through exposure, questioning, purposeful interaction, and identification with a situation that critical thinking skills are developed and enhanced (Lowenstein & Bradshaw, 2001). Examples of learning activities that provide an opportunity to develop critical thinking skills include case studies, clinical scenarios, problem-based learning, discussion, debate, and computer assisted instruction.

There are a number of premier clinical education sites on the Internet that provide excellent opportunities for students to use these techniques in learning clinical skills. The University of Iowa's Virtual Hospital (*http://www.vh.org*), Virtual Children's Hospital (*http://www.vh.org/VCH*), and Virtual Naval Hospital (*http://www.vnh.org*) are among the best and are essential to the education of advance practice nurses. These virtual hospital sites include patient simulations and clinical scenarios from a variety of populations and practice settings. They provide an opportunity for students or practicing APNs to challenge their knowledge on virtually any clinical topic. Working with these simulations provides an opportunity to review assessment, diagnostic reasoning, planning, and evaluation.

The virtual hospital sites, as well as other academic sites such as the University of California at San Francisco's Nurseweb (*http://nurseweb.ucsf.edu/www/arwwebpg.htm*), include links to many primary care sites that provide practice in clinical application of advanced practice knowledge. Encouraging students to develop skill in using these educational sites while in school will also provide them with resources for postgraduate review and expansion of their knowledge, skills, and abilities in clinical practice. The UCSF site was developed by an APN student and it is an excellent site to use in teaching advanced practice nurses (Bliss & DeYoung, 2002). (Please see Fitzpatrick & Montgomery [2000] and Fitzpatrick, Romano, & Chasek [2001] for additional information on Internet sites for health care providers and consumers.)

Assessment skills are fundamental to providing quality health care at all levels of nursing practice. Teaching these skills in an environment devoid of actual examples of normal versus abnormal physical findings creates a challenge for faculty. Assessment courses delivered in both traditional classroom and Web-based environments become a richer experience for students if accompanied by the sights, sounds, and activities that solidify the concepts being presented. Web technology allows for interactivity that includes performing exam procedures on virtual clients with simulated problems. An excellent example of the potential of the Internet in teaching assessment is the University of California at Davis virtual patient site, which includes an eye simulator, pupil response simulator, and patient cases (*http://cim.ucdavis.edu/ Eyes/eyesim.htm*). This Web site provides an opportunity for students to practice examining the eye while viewing how the exam would look in clients with a number of disorders. The student is able to control eye movement as well as the cranial nerves that innervate the muscle in order to simulate clinical situations. The site also provides an interactive quiz after the exam is completed that tests comprehension of the content.

There are numerous sites on the Internet that provide this same interactivity for examining other systems of the body. Realistic lung and heart sounds can be found on sites such as The R.A.L.E Repository Web site (*http://www.rale.ca/*) and the Auscultation Assistant at UCLA (*http://www.wilkes.med.ucla.edu/intro.html*). These sites can be used in the classroom setting as computer assisted instruction or as practice assignments for individual students. The simulators create realistic representations of the normal versus abnormal exam in ways that are not possible in a traditional classroom setting. Interactive exchange improves retention of information whether the instructor is real or virtual (Bastable, 1997).

Advanced practice nurses all have some responsibility for the safe and efficacious use of medication. Medication prescription, administration, and monitoring of responses are common in most practice settings. New medications are being manufactured at a rate that exceeds the ability of pharmacology books to keep up with them. By the time a text or reference book makes it through the editing, publishing, and sales process, new drugs have been added to the repertoire. Rapid access to the information on new drugs has been improved with the advent of the Internet. It is possible to get the latest information at a variety of excellent and timely drug sites including the Physicians' Desk Reference Online Web site (*http://www.pdr.net/*). Directories of medications as well as homepages for the drug companies can be located using any of the popular metasearch engines (please see Montgomery & Uysal [2000] & Montgomery [2001] for more detailed information on drug sites).

In educating students for clinical practice, it is important to include other Internet applications for direct care situations. These include, but are not limited to, the ability to communicate synchronously or asynchronously with patients and colleagues, the ability to monitor clients at a distance (Boyd, 2001; Heldenreich & Ruggerio, 1999), the availability of support groups for virtually any health condition, the presence of clinical practice guidelines (see chapter 1 for additional information on practice guidelines), protocols and current clinical research trials, and the vast number of patient education sites that are maintained by credible organizations (Please see the chapter by Montgomery in this text for additional information on using the Internet in patient education, and Fitzpatrick, Romano, and Chasek [2001] for more information on quality consumer health Web sites). If advanced practice faculty and nurses do not regularly use the Internet in their day-to-day clinical practice they are not maximizing their potential for providing the highest quality of care.

Educator

Nurses throughout the health care system provide information and education. This may be formal education for patients, families, or other health care providers. It may also be education that is informal and provided throughout the day to a variety of contacts. Nurses are asked for advice in virtually every setting they find themselves, whether professional, personal, or social. The advent of the Internet has provided the ability to gather data efficiently on any topic of interest. The Internet can also be used as a resource to refer others to when they are seeking information that the nurse may not have readily available.

The use of the Internet in formal educational environments is being made easier by the installation of "smart classrooms" which allow high-speed Internet access and projection onto a screen. With continuous, reliable high-speed Internet access it is possible to use the Internet interactively in the classroom setting. Graphics on the Internet can be used in conjunction with a Socratic questioning approach to stimulate critical thinking and knowledge applications.

User-friendly point and click Web page development software has made it possible for nurses with limited computer skills to provide information in a Web-based format. This may include syllabi for formal courses, lecture materials, audio and video clips, or simply links to sites that have the desired information. Entrepreneurial advanced practice nurses have used the web to provide client education and updates in their areas of expertise. Web page development for the dissemination of information is rapidly becoming part of graduate education for nurses.

Fully Web-based education and training programs are becoming increasingly common. Nurses can complete much of their advanced practice education without commuting to campus and without disruption of their work life. Across the United States, major universities are adding Web-based options to their graduate programs in advanced practice nursing. Certification and review courses are being offered or developed in most specialty areas. As these options increase, advanced practice nurses in rural settings will be able to more easily continue their education after graduation.

Informal or consumer education is a major function of the Internet. There are thousands of health-related Web sites that can be used. Healthfinder (*http://www.healthfinder.gov*), a site developed by the U.S. Department of Health and Human Services, represents the gold standard in consumer information. This site is user friendly for the novice Web surfer and also is available in Spanish. Other useful consumer sites for client referral include MEDLINEplus at the National Library of Medicine (*http://www.medlineplus.gov/*) and Oncolink at the University of Pennsylvania (*http://cancer.med.upenn.edu/*) for clients wanting information specifically about cancer. The number and variety of Internet sites available for consumer and professional education necessitates that both faculty and students develop a system of cataloging, bookmarking and storing useful annotated links in folders early in their career. This organization of information is a skill that cannot be learned too early in the advanced practice nursing curriculum. In addition, several Internet resource books are available from the editors of this text. (Please see Fitzpatrick and Montgomery [2000] and Fitzpatrick, Romano, and Chasek [2001] for additional information or *http://www.springerpub.com.*)

Researcher

The roles of the advanced practice nurse are well established within the current health care system. In order for these roles to continue to flourish, the measurement of outcomes in advanced practice becomes a mandate (Kleinpell, 2001). Practice-level outcome studies are indicated to document the effect of APN care. Knowledge and use of the research process are essential to measure and document outcomes. The Internet has streamlined the research process by making literature searches readily available. Many research tools are readily available on the Internet at no charge or for nominal fees. Introducing students to these resources early in their course of study teaches them tools to use as they begin practice. (Please see the chapter on research by Belcher and Holdcraft in this text for additional information).

University libraries frequently allow electronic library access for their alumni and current students. Faculty should be aware of the options offered by their own university and encourage students to use these resources while in graduate school. The digitalization of university and private libraries has opened many doors on the Internet. The Virginia Henderson International Nursing Library at the Sigma Theta Tau International Honor Society of Nursing (*http://www.stti.iupui.edu/library/index.html*) is one example of an electronic library available to nurses. All nurses may access many of the library's services; others are available only by subscription. This repository maintains a current registry of nursing research, literature indexes, knowledge bases, and the Online Journal of Knowledge Synthesis for Nursing (OJKSN).

The usefulness of the National Library of Medicine Web site (*http://www.nlm.nih.gov/*) cannot be overstated for the advanced practice nurse. This site allows the nurse to search MEDLINE/PubMed (*http://www.ncbi.nlm.nih.gov/entrez/query.fcgi*), which provides access to over 11 million citations. PubMed provides links to a number of sites that have full-text journal articles. These tools provide powerful resources to support advanced practice research.

In addition to the government sites that provide services at no charge, there are a number of commercial Internet sites that enhance research capabilities on the Web for a fee. The CINAHL (Cumulative Index of Nursing and Allied Health Literature) Web site (*http://www.cinahl.com/*) is among the most useful for advanced practice students. The CINAHL database continues to add titles on a regular basis and currently indexes over 1,200 active journal titles. It is possible to obtain copies of articles electronically or by means of fax through the CINAHL Web site. Web sites such as CINAHL provide cost-effective options for nurse researchers that have limited access to extensive medical libraries. In addition, many university and tertiary care medical centers purchase access to CINAHL for their employees and students.

The nurse researcher can use the Web to communicate with other professionals with similar interests through listservs, newsgroups, and e-mail. A number of professional sites provide forums for discussion of advanced practice issues and trends as well as clinical updates (e.g., Nursingcenter.com at *http://www.nursingcenter.com*). Students should be encouraged to participate in these discussions to enhance learning and socialization to their new advanced practice role. As high-speed Internet access becomes readily available to increasing numbers of practicing nurses, this function will increase in value. Advanced practice nurses are able to collaborate with colleagues for information sharing and support regardless of their geographic location. This creates opportunities that have not previously existed for new graduates as they move into remote practices.

Manager, Leader, and Consultant

Advanced education typically means increased responsibility and opportunities to manage personnel and care. Consultation with other care providers is one expectation of these advanced roles. With the rapid increase in knowledge generation and the volumes of available health care information it is a challenge to maintain currency in one's own field of practice. Technology has been a source of information overload in the practice setting, but also has become part of the solution to the problem. Technology allows us to have voluminous information available at our fingertips. This instant access to information makes it possible to do our jobs well without depending solely on our own memory.

The use of hand-held personal digital devices or assistants for nurses, nurse managers, and consultants is rapidly becoming the norm. These devices include an address and phone book, a to-do list, e-mail, a calculator, a calendar, and the ability to add large amounts of individualized information to the resident memory. With these new systems it is possible for students, faculty, and practitioners to have a personalized virtual library in their pockets. The Internet support of these devices makes it possible to update software and information in minutes. Web sites of interest to advanced practice nurses include PDA Cortex (*http://www.rnpalm.com/*), HandheldMed (*http://www. handheldmed.com/*), Epocrates (*http://www.epocrates.com/*), and e-Medtools (*http://www.e-medtools.com/*). There are many more Web sites supporting personal digital assistants for health care providers and they are programmed to use any of the Internet metasearch engines.

Coding and documentation is of concern to advanced practice nurse managers in all settings. The Web is a rich resource for information on coding and documentation of patient care. Coding manuals are downloadable from a variety of Web sites with links that provide answers to coding and documentation questions. Examples of sites with useful information on coding and documentation are the American Academy of Family Physicians Web site (*http://www.aafp.org/fpm/ medicare/toolbox.html*) and the eMDs (*www.e-mds.com/icd9/index. html*) site, which includes searching capabilities for the International Classification of Diseases (ICD-9).

Advanced practice nurses have been among the nursing leaders who have had an impact on the political process in the United States. One example of this impact has been the passing of legislation that grants prescriptive authority for APNs in a number of states across the nation. Political involvement is critical to the future of both advance practice nursing and quality health care for all. The Internet has facilitated political involvement by creating immediate access to ongoing legislation and communication capabilities with politicians at the state and national level. The American Nurses Association's Government Affairs and Capitol Wiz site (*http://www.nursingworld.org/gova/ state_v1.htm*) allows for fast identification and communication with senators and representatives. This Web site also tracks legislative efforts that are specific to advanced practice registered nurses (APRNs). All APNs should become competent in using such a site during their educational program.

LIMITATIONS AND WEAKNESSES OF USING THE INTERNET IN APN EDUCATION

The Internet is arguably the most powerful and useful tool invented to date for information access in health care. However, as with most great inventions, it has limitations and drawbacks. Having knowledge of the limitations and weaknesses of the system is as important as knowing its value. The limitations of the Internet are primarily a function of hardware, software, infrastructure, vastness, and the ability of anyone to create Web sites without restrictions or standards.

Most Internet sites use graphics as well as audio and video files to increase the power of the information source. As these enhancements are added to Web sites, the speed of access and surfing can be slowed for many users, making the Internet a frustrating and inefficient experience. The speed and usability of the Web is a function of the computer specifications, modem capability, and phone line or cable bandwidth. Any or all of these can make regular use of the Internet impossible due to the time it takes to locate and download Web sites and desired information.

The two most commonly used browsers, Netscape Navigator and Internet Explorer, both read and properly display the Web sites that are most commonly used by advanced practice nurses. However, interactive Web sites may require additional plug-and-play software. As a rule, this additional software can be downloaded from the Web at no charge. The only difficulty with the addition of software is that it uses additional memory, which can become an issue if the computer's memory is limited. If students are asked to visit sites that they cannot access due to hardware or software problems, they may become disheartened with the Internet and unable to recognize its usefulness.

Internet users can also become overwhelmed with the vastness of the Web. Students frequently complain of getting lost when they begin looking for information. They are either unable to locate the information they want, or they find so much information they are not able to sort out what is useful and what is not. Guiding students toward resources for using the Web successfully early in their studies can cut down on their frustration. It is helpful for faculty to provide the best and most applicable sites to students so that they will be successful early in the process. This can be easily achieved with printed handouts of sites, a floppy disk with bookmarks, or a course homepage with links to the desired sites. These same approaches can be recommended to students for later use in sending patients and their families to the Web for information.

The most troubling issue surrounding Internet usage in health care for faculty, clinicians, and patients is the that fact that anyone can create a Web site and provide any information they choose. This results in wide variations in the quality and integrity of health care sites. Education of students and clients must include guidelines for the evaluation of health related Web sites. There are many good tools for Web site evaluation available through educational sites on the Web. The Delaware Academy of Medicine is one example of a site which is devoted to providing accurate information to clients and providers (*http://www.delamed.org/chlsweblinks.html*). As a part of this mission, it provides a variety of mechanisms to ensure that chosen sites carry some assurance that they are reliable and scientifically sound. This site also includes many resources that have already been evaluated by the organization. Providing such a site to students and patients gives them tools for safe and informed use of information available on the Web. (For more information, please see the section by McHugh in this text on cautions for Internet use or Romano and colleagues [2000].)

While the Internet is an excellent information source for faculty and students, it cannot be the only source of information. Overdependence on the Internet can result from the ease of Internet access and use. It is important to reiterate that the Internet is only one source of information. It should not replace the library or other information sources. Use of the Internet alone for education, research, and practice will result in major gaps in knowledge and information. We are not at the point where a hundred percent of what we need to know can be found on the Internet. The necessity for students, faculty, and consumers to use the library cannot be considered dispensable.

The absence of a physical presence when interacting on the Web must also be considered as a potential limitation as education and health care moves toward technology-based delivery systems. The Internet does not currently allow for the reading of nonverbal cues or the use of physical touch. These are important aspects of communication in both education and health care. Although the Internet provides a means of communication, a method of interactivity, and an abundance of resources, it has not yet reached the level of sophistication that would eliminate the need for a human presence in education or health care.

FUTURE DIRECTIONS

Ten years ago it would have been hard to imagine all that is available today over the Internet. The future of technology promises equally dramatic changes in the field of health care over the next decade. Students and faculty will have opportunities to work together to learn and apply the newest technologies in the classroom and clinical setting. Advanced practice nursing will include regular Internet use in areas such as individualized personal Web pages accessible by patient and care providers, links to information on the latest treatment options, and research on the impact of new technologies on health. Health care workers will increasingly be asked to provide health care at a distance using current and new technologies. Web sites for clinical practice will become the standard. The use of the Internet in clinical practice, education, research, management, and consulting will be required if advanced practice nurses are to continue to provide the highest quality of health care in the new millennium.

WEB SITE RECAP

American Academy of Family Physicians
http://www.aafp.org/fpm/medicare/toolbox.html

American Nurses Association Capitol Wiz
http://www.nursingworld.org/gova/state_v1.htm

Auscultation Assistant at UCLA
http://www.wilkes.med.ucla.edu/intro.html

Cumulative Index of Nursing and Allied Health Literature (CINAHL)
http://www.cinahl.com/

Delaware Academy of Medicine
http://www.delamed.org/chlsweblinks.html

eMDs
http://www.e-mds.com/icd9/index.html

e-Medtools
http://www.e-medtools.com/

Epocrates
http://www.epocrates.com/

Eye Simulator
http://cim.ucdavis.edu/eyes/eyesim.htm

HandheldMed
http://www.handheldmed.com/

Healthfinder
http://www.healthfinder.gov

MEDLINE/PubMed
http://www.ncbi.nlm.nih.gov/entrez/query.fcgi

MEDLINEplus at the National Library of Medicine
http://www.medlineplus.gov/

Nursingcenter.com
http://www.nursingcenter.com

Oncolink at the University of Pennsylvania
http://cancer.med.upenn.edu/

PDA Cortex
http://www.rnpalm.com/

Physicians' Desk Reference Online
http://www.pdr.net/

Springer Publishing Company
http://www.springerpub.com

The R.A.L.E Repository Web site
http://www.rale.ca/

The Virginia Henderson International Nursing Library
http://www.stti.iupui.edu/library/index.html

UCSF Nurseweb
http://nurseweb.ucsf.edu/www/arwwebpg.htm

University of Iowa's Virtual Hospital
http://www.vh.org

Virtual Children's Hospital
http://www.vh.org/VCH

Virtual Naval Hospital
http://www.vnh.org

REFERENCES

Bastable, S. B. (1997). *Nurse as educator: Principles of teaching and learning.* Boston: Jones and Bartlett.

Bauer, J. C., & Ringel, M. A. (1999). *Telemedicine and the reinvention of health care.* New York: McGraw Hill.

Berger, A. M., Eilers, J. G., Pattrin, L., Rolf-Fixley, M., Pfeifer, B. A., Rogge, J. A., Wheeler, L. M., Bergstrom, N. I., & Heck, C. S. (1996). Advanced practice roles for nurses in tomorrow's healthcare systems. *Clinical Nurse Specialist, 10,* 250–255.

Bliss, J. B., & DeYoung, S. (2002). *Working the Web: A guide for nurses.* Upper Saddle River, NJ: Prentice Hall.

Boyd, L. (2001). Monitoring patients. *RN, 64*(2), 53–54.

Carty, B. (Ed.). (2000). *Nursing informatics: Education for practice.* New York: Springer Publishing Co.

Fitzpatrick, J. J., & Montgomery, K. S. (Eds.). (2000). *Internet resources for nurses.* New York: Springer Publishing Co.

Fitzpatrick, J. J., Romano, C., & Chasek, R. (Eds.). (2001). *The nurses' guide to consumer health Web sites.* New York: Springer Publishing Co.

Heidenreich, P., & Ruggerio, C. (1999). Effect of a home monitoring system on hospitalization and resource use for patients with heart failure. *American Heart Journal, 138*(4), 633.

Kleinpell, R. M. (Ed.) (2001). *Outcome assessment in advanced practice nursing.* New York: Springer Publishing Co.

Lowenstein, A. J., & Bradshaw, M. J. (2001). *Fuszard's innovative teaching strategies in nursing.* Gaithersburg, MD: Aspen.

Montgomery, K. S. (2001). Drug information and medications. In J. J. Fitzpatrick, C. Romano, & R. Chasek (Eds.), *The nurses' guide to consumer health Web sites* (pp. 15–19). New York: Springer Publishing Co.

Montgomery, K. S., & Uysal, A. (2000). Pharmaceutical resources. In J. J. Fitzpatrick & K. S. Montgomery (Eds.), *Internet resources for nurses* (pp. 10–16). New York: Springer Publishing Co.

Romano, C. A., Hinegardner, P. G., & Phyillaier, C. R. (2000). Consumer health resources. In J. J. Fitzpatrick & K. S. Montgomery (Eds.), *Internet resources for nurses* (pp. 17–29). New York: Springer Publishing Co.

Chapter 14

Benchmarks for Successful Internet-Based Education

Carol Pullen

There has been considerable controversy surrounding the quality of online learning and the feasibility of online learning for RNs. A study produced by The Institute for Higher Education Policy (IHEP) identified 24 benchmarks considered essential to ensuring excellence in Internet-based distance education (IHEP, 2000). The benchmarks are divided into seven categories of quality measures currently in use at six institutions recognized as leaders in distance education. These benchmarks were identified to help policymakers, faculty, and students in making sound decisions about the quality of online learning. There are many student issues associated with learning via the Internet. The benchmarks pertaining to students will be used as an organizing framework for this chapter. Twelve benchmarks in four different categories appear to have the most relevance for RN students. These benchmarks will assist faculty in designing and implementing quality online programs. RN students can use these benchmarks to make decisions about choosing an online program.

COURSE DEVELOPMENT BENCHMARKS

One of the three course development benchmarks pertains to student issues around course design. According to the IHEP study (2000, p. 2), **"Courses are designed to require students to engage them-**

selves in analysis, synthesis, and evaluation as part of their course and program requirements." Two major objectives for RNs in BSN programs are to a) master problem solving and critical thinking skills needed for professional clinical decision-making and b) become socialized to the role of the professional nurse. These skills and role changes can be taught and facilitated in online courses.

In online courses, faculty can help RN students develop critical thinking skills by shifting from the instructor paradigm prevalent in much of today's education to a student-centered learning paradigm, where the focus is shifted from instruction to learning (Van Dusen, 1997). A student-centered learning model promotes self-discipline and requires students to take more responsibility for their learning (Yeaworth, Pullen, Zimmerman, & Hays, 2001). RN students are well suited to a student-centered model, according to Krouse (1988), who found that RN students are likely to be mature and independent learners.

As Alley (1996) put it:

> If a sage on a stage is the metaphor for traditional passive learning environments, then learner on stage and support staff as stage hands, with professor directing it all is a metaphor for the student-centered learning we want to achieve. (p. 51)

RN students bring a wealth of knowledge and experience to the classroom; it is important to help them use these strengths for greater learning to take place. Palloff and Pratt (2001) propose that students have three main roles in online learning, that is, knowledge generation, collaboration, and process management. The term knowledge generation implies that students construct their own meaning of knowledge by analyzing material critically and presenting it to their classmates and faculty. This is one method for RNs to demonstrate their critical thinking skills. Collaboration is a skill that most RNs have developed by working collaboratively with other health care professionals. Students should be given assignments that promote and require online collaboration, and one aspect of collaboration is to share knowledge and resources with other students. Online student discussions can lead to a deeper level of understanding as students propose different views and evaluate the material with group input. Only a few students actually attain process management, and they become group leaders who create new boundaries for students and faculty. Faculty must be cognizant of these emerging roles and willing to let the process occur. According to Krouse's study (1988), beginning RN students show leadership potential, and many students may be seeking opportunities to develop these skills.

RN students who were educated in traditional environments such as diploma or associate degree programs may need assistance with their roles in online education. Palloff and Pratt (2001) noted that the use of technology had a significant impact on the learning process itself and that learning online is more than attaining competence with the hardware and software. They also suggested that faculty can teach their students to use the online environment more effectively. RN students actually need to be made aware of the changing roles of instructor and student to help them be comfortable and successful in this new environment. A period of transition may be necessary to help students adopt a student-centered paradigm of learning. This is important for RN students as many of them are also making the role transition to student while trying to successfully balance the demands of their jobs, families, and educational programs.

Socialization to the profession by RN students is defined by Wooley (1978) as "a whole behavioral change—in their attitudes, role, and functions" (p.103). The process of socialization is facilitated by the academic environment, which provides frequent interaction with faculty and students, availability of scholarly resources, and exposure to a variety of new ideas and experiences (Cragg, 1991). Internet-based education does limit the amount of face-to-face contact RN students will have with faculty and with each other. However, socialization of the RN can be accomplished using the vast array of online resources and by incorporating online modules that require faculty and student interaction. In a qualitative study with 24 RN students at four universities, students engaged in either group teleconferences or individualized correspondence courses, and answered questions via a telephone interview (Cragg). The results showed that both methods in these distance education courses were influential in the professional socialization of RN students. In a study of 219 RN students enrolled in online courses at three schools of nursing, students reported socialization as an outcome of the courses (Billings, Connors, & Skiba, 2001). Further exploration of socialization outcomes for RN students engaged in Internet-based education are needed.

TEACHING/LEARNING BENCHMARKS

The three teaching/learning benchmarks with direct relevance to RN students address interaction, feedback, and effective research.

Student Interaction

According to the IHEP study (2000, p. 2), **"Student interaction with faculty and other students is an essential characteristic. . . . "** Internet-based education uses a variety of synchronous (real time) and asynchronous (not real time) methods to promote interactivity. Synchronous methods include text-based methods such as scheduled chat rooms and "instant messenger" features for immediate access. Another synchronous method is desktop videoconferencing that incorporates audio, video, and print delivery via a desktop computer, a camera, and software, such as Cu-SeeMe, developed at Cornell University. The most frequently used asynchronous methods are e-mail, case studies, group discussions, and collaborative projects.

Students often complain of feeling isolated and unconnected when they use distance learning technologies (Hill, 1997). But, Cragg (1994) found that RN students reported that computer conferencing decreased isolation since they had a sense of someone always being there for them. Nevertheless, students indicated that some form of face-to-face interaction was helpful. Student surveys have shown a high level of satisfaction and better learning outcomes when there is a high level of interaction with classmates and high levels of participation in the courses (Hiltz, 2001). In addition, interaction with class members in chat rooms and discussion groups establishes an important foundation for collaborative team building (O'Brien & Renner, 2000). According to Niederhauser, Bigley, Hale, and Harper (1999) faculty observed a sense of independence, empowerment, and creativity as RN students took control of the discussion groups. In addition, Hiltz (2001) recommended using software that provides a private area for student group work. Student lounges without faculty access can be set up on Web sites to allow students to socialize on line. Students indicate that they like using the Internet to communicate with each other since phone costs for interaction can be prohibitive.

Palloff and Pratt (2001) noted: "Successful learners in the online environment need to be active, creative, and engaged in the learning process" (p. 107). Students who do not participate as freely in discussions in the traditional classroom may flourish in asynchronous discussions because of the time for reflection before responding. Interactive skills learned in the online environment may carry over to face-to-face settings. RN students in an online distance education seminar become more self-directed. Furthermore, even those students, whose class participation was only minimal, posted thought-provoking and persua-sive arguments (Albrekton, 1995). Faculty must be actively involved in guiding students if they stray from the learning objectives and in resolving conflicts that may arise. Billings and colleagues (2001) found that isolation of students is negatively correlated to course satisfaction and interactivity is critical to reducing isolation.

Student feedback. **Constructive and timely feedback should be provided to students** (IHEP, 2000).

> Probably the single most important behavioral practice, which produces relatively good results in online courses, is the timely and personal (in tone) response by instructors to questions and contributions of student online. (Hiltz, 1995, p. 8)

Most RNs are motivated and committed to performing well in school. They want to know if they are meeting the course objectives and, specifically, what their grades are. At the beginning of the course, faculty can establish guidelines on feedback, such as how often the student should expect feedback and what type of feedback will be provided. Faculty may post online frequently and be an active partici-pant in the discussion, or faculty may set up more student-centered discussions and participate as needed to redirect the discussion or to provide positive feedback. Feedback can be e-mailed directly to individual students and/or to the group as a whole. Helping students provide feedback to other learners enhances the overall interactivity (Rasmussen, Northrup, & Lee, 1997). Initially, students may be reluc-tant to challenge other students or to give feedback. Faculty can serve as a role model and provide guidance on effective ways to give feed-back.

Effective Research

According to the IHEP study (2000, p. 3), **"Students are instructed in the proper methods of effective research, including assessment of the validity of resources."** RN students will need assistance in learning about the many resources of the Internet and how best to search for the information they need. Older students sometimes say that they first learned about the resources of the Internet from their children, and many have not fully used the Internet for their own personal uses. Novices to the Internet may have difficult assessing the validity and usefulness of an Internet site. Rakes (1996) recommends initial steps that faculty should take in implementing what he describes as "resource-based learning." He suggested that faculty pose a question or problem, provide a range of universal resource locators (URLs), and evaluate the process that was used to determine if the learning objective was met. The development of these skills will help the RN student throughout the program and they will also be better able to access and evaluate information needed for their nursing practice.

COURSE STRUCTURE BENCHMARKS

All five course structure benchmarks are important considerations for RN students prior to entering, and during, a distance education program.

Advisement Process

RN students should be advised prior to starting a distance education program about the nature of the program (IHEP, 2000). Advisers should be prepared to discuss the differences in online and traditional learning in nursing programs and the options available to the students. Online learning may not be the best choice for students who require a great deal of structure and who cannot work independently. However, most RN students are motivated, self-disciplined, and willing to make the commitment to a course format that requires more independent and collaborative learning, particularly if they are unable to access courses by traditional means. Students must be informed as to the software and hardware required for participation in the online program. It is helpful to provide information about the various Internet services available and how the Internet service impacts the course delivery. Students in rural areas may only have access to dial-in services with very narrow bandwidth, thus necessitating longer times to download content. Some programs supplement online courses with CD-ROM technology to decrease the amount of online time, but an additional fee may be assessed for this service.

Supplemental Course Information

Students should be provided with supplemental course information that includes course objectives and learning outcomes that are summarized clearly (IHEP, 2000). RN programs typically have very detailed syllabi and accrediting bodies require clear course objectives and learning outcomes. This information may be placed online, but faculty should place the entire syllabus in a folder or under a button for students to print. Busy RN students often complain that course information and course content are overlooked, since material is often placed in online areas not readily identifiable to the student. Initially, print copies of the syllabus or course packets may be provided to assist the students in their transition to the online world of education.

Library Resources

Students should have access to adequate library resources (IHEP, 2000). Luther (1998) emphasizes that distance education students must have corresponding resources available to them in an easily accessible digital format from the library. Some libraries now have a "virtual library" with their resources available through the World Wide Web. Library portals are the wave of the future as libraries are looking for a more customized consumer-centered approach (Buchanan, 2001).

At the University of Nebraska Medical Center, the McGoogan Library and the College of Nursing conducted a pilot project to demonstrate the feasibility of electronic access to articles in two nursing courses (Reidelbach & Pullen, 2000). Copyright permission was granted either from the Copyright Clearance Center or directly from the publisher. Unfortunately, many publishing companies would not grant copyright permission to digitize and place articles online and consequently permission was received for only one-half to two-thirds of the articles in the two courses. Students indicated that they were satisfied with this method of obtaining course readings, but some students complained that the time required to download articles was excessive. This was particularly true for students with slower computer processors, or for students living in more remote areas with only narrow bandwidth available from Internet service providers. It will be helpful to nursing students when libraries subscribe to more electronic journals. In the interim, packets of course readings or a combination of course packets, digitized articles, and electronic journals may be the best option.

FACULTY AND STUDENT EXPECTATIONS

According to the IHEP study, **"Faculty and students should agree upon expectations regarding times for student assignment completion and faculty response"** (2000, p. 3). At the beginning of online learning, students need more structure. RN students, busy with family and work responsibilities, appreciate clear guidelines as to what is expected in a course and like to be involved in decisions as to when assignments are due. Faculty may want to allow some initial flexibility if students do not have assignments in on time. If late submissions become a recurring problem, it will be necessary to assess students' technology skills and/or study habits. Online students also want feedback in a timely manner. Therefore, faculty should tell students when to expect a response to their submissions. Some faculty have tried posting virtual office hours in order to be available at specific times to students. Another option is to post hours for phone consultations.

Student Support Benchmarks

Four benchmarks address support for students in obtaining program information, resource retrieval, technical assistance, and developing a system to handle complaints or questions.

Program Information

"Students receive information about programs, including admission requirements, tuition and fees, books and supplies, technical and proctoring requirements, and student support services" (IHEP, 2000, p. 3). Online students should receive the same information that is provided to other RN students. Additional information may be provided for online students if requirements or services differ, such as computer requirements and troubleshooting support for technical questions. If students are taking the courses from a distance, many schools use proctors for either print or online tests. Proctors should be identified at the beginning of the program and given an introduction to their expectations. The College of Nursing at the University of Nebraska Medical Center uses a form letter that explains the role of the proctor and the role of the college in student testing. Guidelines for online testing have been developed. Print copies of tests are mailed to proctors in the event there is a problem administering the online test.

Resource Retrieval

"Students are provided with hands-on training and information to aid them in securing material through electronic databases, interlibrary loans, government archives, news services, and other sources" (IHEP, 2000, p. 3). Throughout an online program, RN students will be introduced to the rich resources of the Internet. Initial and ongoing instruction will be necessary to ensure that they can secure relevant material in a timely manner. RN students not familiar with the Internet can waste valuable time if they do not know how to properly search for the information they need.

Technical Assistance

Students should have access to technical assistance beginning with a detailed orientation, practice sessions, and ongoing access to technical support staff (IHEP, 2000, p. 3). Researchers have found that technical support with a help desk is essential for satisfied and successful online RN students (O'Brien & Renner, 2000). RN students often do not have a great deal of experience with computers or online activities. Some students who work in settings where computers are used may have computer skills, but often not the skills needed for online learning. Although troubleshooting computer problems throughout the student's course of study is the responsibility of the technical support staff, RN students need to learn many computer skills up front. Skills such as word processing, using spreadsheets and databases, using the institutions' e-mail system, conducting library and Internet searches, downloading and installing software both from a disc and from the Internet, learning to use the course software such as Blackboard or a "home grown" system, and posting to discussion groups are the most common skills needed. Appropriate communication skills for online learning should be included in an orientation to the program. The acquisition of technical skills may be required prior to program entry by completion of a required orientation or a computer course, or offered in the first course or later courses when needed in the program. A combination of these methods may be employed. Students may be assigned certain technical skills to complete at the beginning of a course to ensure that they have the necessary skills. Examples may be sending an e-mail, downloading free software from the Internet, locating URLs from credible Web sites pertinent to a particular topic, and/or participating in an online discussion.

Many online nursing programs are unprepared to provide the level of technical support necessary to support students anywhere, anytime. The most problematic area is providing the ideal 24-hour-a-day, 7-day-week support for students who will be accessing coursework at times most convenient to them. Outsourcing of technical support is a possibility, but that may be an expensive solution. Collaboration with the college or university's information technology department may be helpful to provide the support. A variety of methods may be used to provide technical support. Phone contact is the most expensive method, but preferred by many RN students due to the immediate access and opportunity to talk directly to an expert. Other methods, such as using a pager system to contact on-call personnel, sending an e-mail, or faxing questions are viable options to consider. Written or online handouts can provide answers to frequently asked questions and assist students in problem solving their own technical problems. Some questions are more appropriately addressed to the local Internet service provider or even to the company from which the student purchased the computer. At Old Dominion University, RN students are required to complete a computer checklist developed by computer services and present compatibility information when help is needed (Benjamin-Coleman, Smith, Alexy, & Palmer, 2001).

Regardless of the method of support available to the student, students should receive adequate information about the expected response time. For example, e-mail support may be provided within a 24-hour period. Students will need to plan, at least initially, extra time to be sure they have mastered the technology that is required for the submission of an assignment. A proactive approach to troubleshooting may be the most effective. One very simple solution to technical difficulties on a weekend or evening when the assignment is due on Monday or early the next day is to have assignments due later in the week or during the day. This approach will give the support staff time to respond to the student and correct the problem if needed. It may not be possible to correct problems on the weekend or in the evening.

A backup plan should always be in place for any type of online class delivery. For synchronous classes, materials may be sent prior to class via e-mail in case the video system fails during a scheduled class session. Telephone can be used if there are audio problems. Telephone bridges should be set up prior to the class with the number to call if needed. Synchronous chats can be archived for later review by students who cannot connect. For students attempting to complete assignments or send materials to faculty, they should be advised that they could fax or mail assignments if difficulty arises.

System for Student Questions and Concerns

A structured system should be in place to address student concerns. Student service personnel should respond accurately and quickly to questions (IHEP, 2000). A solid infrastructure for distance education should be in place to ensure that online RN students have access to the same services as students on campus who can resolve questions by visiting the relevant office. Online students have to learn other methods to obtain support such as phone, e-mail, or fax. Ideally, online students have a single person they can contact for all administrative problems or at least one person who directs them to the proper resource. Initially, online students may require greater assistance, since they may feel more isolated. On campus students get information from other students. An online site designed specifically for student interaction may promote more informal opportunities for information sharing among students.

STUDENT EVALUATION OF ONLINE COURSES

Ongoing evaluation of RN Internet-based educational programs, using both formative and summative methods, is essential to further understand student issues and to make adjustments to ensure student satisfaction and a quality online program. Administrators and faculty must be attuned to students needs and comments throughout the program. The needs of RN students may be different from other student groups, and their input is critical. At least three student surveys, such as evaluations of the course, evaluations of the faculty, and evaluations of the technology, should be used for each course, every semester. Students should have the opportunity to provide written comments on each evaluation form. A rich, but time-consuming method of evaluation, is the use of focus groups to allow students the opportunity to express both positive and negative experiences in online education. Focus groups allow the evaluator to observe student growth throughout the program and that is helpful feedback to faculty as they continue to revise the program and courses. Additional information must be kept about online students' questions and problems, including technical support logs that document the time and nature of problems and what efforts were needed to resolve them.

CONCLUSIONS

The AACN (1999) proposes consideration of several factors that have implications in order for students to take full advantage of distance education technology. These factors include methods to increase nurses' access to educational programs, measures to ensure privacy of educational dialogue, and enhanced student support structures.

Gilbert, a national leader in the use of technology in higher education, suggests that the new challenge for students could be to learn to take advantage of too many options—instead of too few (2001). The three dimensions of change that he advocates watching are individualization (responding to different learning styles), standardization and access (equitable and convenient access to information resources), and personalization (enhancing communication and "connectedness"). Although these topics have been previously considered in the literature, further exploration and research is needed to determine their influence on quality online education.

Online courses hold much promise for increasing access to baccalaureate education for RNs, who are highly motivated adult learners. Studies have shown that learning outcomes for online courses are positive, and RN students are satisfied with online learning (Billings, Connors, & Skiba, 2001; Halstead & Coudret, 2000; Niederhauser, Bigley, Hale, & Harper, 1999; O'Brien & Renner, 2000; Leasure, Davis, & Thievon, 2000; Ryan, Carlton, & Ali, 1999; Soon, Sook, Jung, & Im, 2000). The opportunities for online learning are almost limitless. Online education transcends time and distance barriers to fully realize learning anywhere, anytime. Course work can now be provided in highly interactive formats including audio, video, and text, and new technologies are emerging to further enhance course delivery. Students will be challenged to master new technologies, but it is conceivable that students may have so many options for their education that they will demand quality online education.

REFERENCES

Albrektson, J. R. (1995). Mentored online seminar: A model for graduate-level distance learning. *T.H.E. Journal, 23*, 102–105.

Alley, L. R. (1996). An instructional epiphany. *Change, 4*, 50–54.

American Association of Colleges of Nursing (1999). *AACN white paper: Distance technology in nursing education*. [Online]. Available: *http://www.aacn.nche.edu/*

Benjamin-Coleman, R., Smith, M., Alexy, B., & Palmer, K. (2001). A decade of distance education: RN to BSN. *Nurse Educator, 26*, 9–12.

Billings, D. M., Connors, H. R., & Skiba, D. J. (2001). Benchmarking best practices in Web-based nursing courses. *Advances in Nursing Science, 23*, 41–52.

Buchanan, E. A. (2001). Ready or not, they're here: Library portals. *Syllabus, 14*(12), 30–31.

Cragg, C. E. (1991). Professional resocialization of post-RN baccalaureate students by distance education. *Journal of Nursing Education, 30*, 256–260.

Cragg, C. E. (1994.) Distance learning through computer conferences. *Nurse Educator, 19*, 10–14.

Gilbert, S. W. (2001). Dimensions of technology change. *Syllabus, 14*(12), 28.

Halstead, J. A., & Coudret, N. A. (2000). Implementing web-based instruction in a school of nursing: Implications for faculty and students. *Journal of Professional Nursing, 16*, 273–281.

Hill, J. R. (1997). Distance learning environments via the World Wide Web. In B. H. Khan (Ed.), *Web-based instruction* (pp. 75–80). Englewood Cliffs, NJ: Educational Technology.

Hiltz, S. R. (1995). Teaching in a virtual classroom. Presented at the 1995 International Conference on Computer Assisted Instruction, Hsinchu, Taiwan. Available: *www.njit.edu/njit/department/cccc/vc/papers/teaching.html*

Hiltz, S. R. (2001). Learning effectiveness. In J. Moore (Ed.), *Online education* (p. 5). Needham, MA: Sloan Center for Online Education.

Institute for Higher Education Policy. (2000). *Quality on the line: Benchmarks for success in Internet-based distance education*. Washington, DC: Author.

Krouse, H. J. (1988). Personality characteristics of registered nurses in baccalaureate education. *Nurse Educator, 13*, 27, 36, 39.

Leasure, A. R., Davis, L., & Thievon, S. L. (2000). Comparison of student outcomes and preferences in a traditional vs. world wide web-based research course. *Journal of Nursing Education, 39*, 149–154.

Luther, J. (1998). Distance learning and the digital library: Or what happens when the virtual student needs to use the virtual library in a virtual university? *Educom Review, 33*, 23–26.

Niederhauser, V. P., Bigley, M. B., Hale, J., & Harper, D. (1999). Cybercases: An innovation in Internet education. *Journal of Nursing Education, 38*, 415–418.

O'Brien, B. S., & Renner, A. (2000). Nurses on-line: Career mobility for registered nurses. *Journal of Professional Nursing, 16*, 16–20.

Palloff, R., & Pratt, K. (2001). *Lessons from the cyberspace classroom: The realities of online teaching*. San Francisco: Jossey-Bass.

Potempa, K., Stanley, J., Davis, B., Miller, K., Hassett, M., & Pepicello, S. (2001). Survey of distance technology use in AACN member schools. *Journal of Professional Nursing, 17*, 7–13.

Rakes, G. C. (1996). Using the Internet as a tool in a resource-based learning environment. *Educational Technology, 36*, 52–56.

Rasmussen, K., Northrup, P., & Lee, R. (1997). Implementing web-based instruction. In B. H. Khan (Ed.), *Web-based instruction* (pp. 341–346). Englewood Cliffs, NJ: Educational Technology.

Reidelbach, M., & Pullen, C. H. (2000). [Electronic reserve service]. Unpublished raw data.

Ribbons, R. (1998). Practical applications in nurse education. *Nurse Education Today, 18*, 413–418.

Ryan, M., Carlton, K. H., & Ali, N. S. (1999). Evaluation of traditional classroom teaching methods versus course delivery via the World Wide Web. *Journal of Nursing Education, 38*, 272–277.

Soon, K. H., Sook, K. I., Jung, C. W., & Im, K. M. (2000). The effects of Internet-based distance learning in nursing. *Computers in Nursing, 18*, 19–25.

Van Dusen, G. C. (1997). *The virtual campus: Technology and reform in higher education*. ASHE-ERIC Higher Education Report Volume 25, No. 5. Washington, DC: George Washington University, Graduate School of Education and Human Development.

Wooley, A. S. (1978). From RN to BSN: Faculty perceptions. *Nursing Outlook, 26*, 103–108.

Yeaworth, R., Pullen, C. H., Zimmerman, L., & Hays, B. (2001). Distributed learning strategies: Improving educational access in nursing. In N. L. Chaska (Ed.), *The nursing profession: Tomorrow and beyond* (pp. 165–175). Thousand Oaks, CA: Sage.

_____ Chapter **15**

Internet Use in the Traditional Classroom

Kristen S. Montgomery

I n the very recent past, nurses have witnessed an explosion in Internet-based distance education. Distance education is not feasible or even desirable for all students, however. This chapter addresses use of the Internet in traditional classroom settings. The Internet can be used to enhance or supplement the traditional classroom environment in several ways. For example, students can look up and evaluate information on Web sites, provide their colleagues with examples of Web sites, highlight strengths and weakness of Web sites, or search for information during a traditional course. Internet-based assignments can be completed in class or outside of class as homework assignments. Each of these areas of opportunity will be addressed in more detail, and the strengths and limitations of these types of assignments will be discussed.

APPLICATIONS OF INTERNET USE IN THE TRADITIONAL CLASSROOM

In the traditional classroom setting, three main applications of the Internet occur: use by faculty to enhance teaching and learning, in-class assignments for students, and homework assignments for students outside of class. Each of these mechanisms for Internet use in the traditional classroom will be discussed.

Faculty Applications

Faculty can integrate the Internet into traditional classroom environments in numerous ways. Use of the Internet can enhance faculty presentations of learning content, faculty can highlight key Web sites for a particular topic area (e.g., nutrition), or faculty can teach skills regarding Internet use. These Internet skills may include evaluating Web sites or how to use the Internet itself. (Please see Romano, Hinegardner, & Phyillaier [2000] and Holloway, Kripps, Koepke, & Skiba [2000] for additional information on evaluating Web sites.)

The Internet can be useful to enhance material presented when there is a quality Web site that can supplement the information provided in class. Web sites often have learning modules, PowerPoint slides, or other material that might enhance the lecture or discussion provided by the faculty member. Online continuing education (CE) courses may also be useful in certain settings. (Please see the chapter on continuing education for additional information.)

Faculty may also highlight key Web sites that are related to the topic of interest. For example, if the topic were nutrition, faculty could highlight the American Dietetics Association Web site (*http://www.eatright.org*) and evaluate the information and layout of the site during the classroom discussion. Additionally, faculty can provide and assist students in critiquing Web sites that are focused on consumers. An example of a Web site on nutrition developed for consumers is: *http://www.foodfit. com*. The faculty member or student could access this site and have it projected onto a large screen for all to see. The class could evaluate the content and layout of the site as part of the classroom discussion. Having such discussions can facilitate other students' learning, since not everyone will identify the same issues if the Web site is viewed individually. (Please see Montgomery [2000] and Morin [2001] for additional information on Web sites related to nutrition.) Discussion of Web sites and using the Internet in class can be facilitated with the use of an LCD projector that displays what the user would normally see on the computer screen to a large screen that facilitates viewing for everyone.

Strengths and Weaknesses of Faculty Applications

Facilitating students' learning and interest by using a wide variety of mediums to deliver course content is one of the strengths of using the

Internet in the traditional classroom. Not all students learn in the same way. Thus, using a variety of sources may help some students to learn better and can also break up the monotony that sometimes occurs when there is overreliance on one method of instruction (e.g., lecture).

Potential disadvantages of using the Internet in this capacity include the need for increased equipment that is often costly and personnel who can help faculty with problems when they arise. CE courses may involve additional costs. In addition, it may be difficult to cover only one module, or to begin the CE course somewhere other than the beginning. Additionally, CE courses or other Web sites may not always work. Planning backup activities in the event a Web site is not functioning on class day can facilitate learning the necessary material. It is also possible to save Web pages to a disk, which could be used in the event the Web site is down at the needed time. Consideration also needs to be given to faculty training to address learning needs on the Internet beyond just repeating what was formerly done on paper (e.g., administration of the same medication test online instead of paper) in order to use the Internet to its full capabilities in the traditional classroom (Collins & Dewees, 2001).

Internet-Based Student Assignments

Internet-based assignments can either be done in class or outside of class. In either case, students often present their work to their colleagues in the course. In-class assignments can include work that is actually done in the classroom or work that is done outside the classroom and then presented to the class as part of course requirements. Outside assignments include student research that is used for another purpose (e.g., literature review using CINAHL or PubMed). Students may work individually or in groups (Poindexter & Basu, 2000). Internet-based student assignments are similar to usage strategies identified for faculty. Some sample assignments include:

- Students search the Internet for quality Web sites on certain topics that are appropriate for nurses or consumers and present these with critique to their classmates,
- Students identify Web sites that teach a particular skill (e.g., cardiac sounds) and present these with critique to their classmates,
- Students identify professional and political resources to assist with a patient-care issue,

- Students or groups of students are assigned a case "family" for the semester for which they identify Web sites that would be appropriate for this family's needs (this is a higher-level assignment since the student needs to assess what the family's needs are and then find Web sites that are appropriate).
- Students can be assigned or choose a university's Web site to evaluate what they perceive to be the benefits and concerns about attending one of their programs based on the information obtained from the Web site (undergraduate students can look at graduate programs and master's students can evaluate doctoral programs). This information can be presented to their colleagues during class time or the search and critique can be done as part of class. This type of assignment will promote student learning regarding the characteristics of graduate programs, how to evaluate such programs, and critique of whether or not a particular school is covering important content. This focuses the student toward the critical issues influencing health care. For example, some key issues that are currently affecting health care in this country include the nursing shortage and health insurance coverage for all citizens. If these are key issues of importance to nurses, the topics ought to be covered in the school's nursing curriculum. Therefore, the student would be expected to identify the lack of a health policy course or content as a significant problem in the educational program. For graduate students who are evaluating doctoral programs, they can evaluate what areas are significant for health care researchers. For example, does the curriculum include instruction in both qualitative and quantitative methods? Are the faculty teaching in the doctoral program funded? Identifying important aspects of the research process is an expected outcome of graduate level research courses.

Strengths and Weaknesses of Internet-Based Student Assignments

Internet-based assignments force those students who have not yet taken advantage of Internet technology to become familiar with its use. Using the Internet is no longer considered a "nice" skill to have, but is rather considered essential in many settings. The necessity of Internet skills will continue to increase in the future. Internet skills are probably most essential for returning RN students who may have been in the practice setting for an extended period of time. This may also be true for some graduate students who have been functioning in practice settings. Undergraduates as a group are much more likely to have Internet skills from high school or other experiences. Nursing is probably one of the last professions to be included in the group of professions that require their members to have expertise in Internet use, since much of their work is done away from a desk, unlike many other professions.

Presentations, Internet-based or otherwise, provide students with experience speaking and responding to questions from small groups. In-class assignments also help to keep class lively and can encourage participation from students. Internet-based assignments are a way to let students shine with the discoveries they can make online.

The basic weaknesses of Internet-based assignments for students are similar to the weaknesses identified for faculty. Essentially, the time and expertise required to maintain the equipment and to problem-solve when complications arise. Cost issues are also a significant concern. Internet-based assignments that students must complete outside of class can increase student burden if they do not have Internet access at their home or dorm. However, Internet access is increasingly available at alternate sites such as the library, and many schools have their own computer labs for students use. Most faculty would probably concur that the value of Internet-based assignments generally outweighs the small amount of student inconvenience.

WEB RESOURCES

A Web search did not reveal any Web sites specific to nurse educators regarding using the Internet in the nursing classroom. There were, however, several sites worthy of mention that were developed for other audiences, but have the potential to be useful to nurse educators. These are listed in the text that follows.

Internet Activities for Foreign Language Classes
http://members.aol.com/maestro12/web/wadir.html

Internet Activities for foreign language classes includes information on writing activities for the Web, reading strategies for the Web, and Internet options in the classroom. One can download and print information for activities. The author of this site also provides helpful information on issues of copyright regarding information printed from the Web and distributed to a class, saving individual Web pages on disk, and links to favorite teacher URLs are provided in Spanish, French, and German. Sample lesson plans are also provided and sorted by language and student level. Although these lesson plans are related to language and generally geared toward younger audiences, they may be useful for students and faculty who are interested in learning another language.

Internet in the Classroom: First Steps
http://home.swbell.net/jraneri/Internetintheclassroom.htm

Internet in the Classroom: First Steps is a list of Web sites for educators. Most of these sites are geared toward K-12 educators, but some of the ideas and principles can also be applied to higher education.

Common Questions About Integrating the Internet into the Classroom
http://www.iloveteaching.com/Intenetclass/index.htm

Common Questions About Integrating the Internet into the Classroom offers informative information on using the Internet to reinforce content and practical applications. Again, this site is mostly geared toward K-12 teachers. However, much of the information provided is applicable to higher education as well.

Using the Internet in the Classroom
http://mason.gmu.edu/~montecin/IDOweb-w.htm

Using the Internet in the Classroom is a good resource for information on assignments that involve student groups critiquing Web sites and presenting to others, and Internet searches for appropriate resources.

Your Internet Guides: Internet Primer
http://www.thirteen.org/edonline/primer

This Internet primer was developed for K–12 teachers who are new to the Internet. The site is well designed and may also be useful to nurses and nurse educators who are new to the Internet.

PRACTICAL CONSIDERATIONS

While there are many benefits to using the Internet in the classroom, the faculty member who wishes to do so, particularly on a regular basis, will also find that using the Internet in the classroom adds some extra burden as well. There is time involved in setting up the equipment and, of course, the equipment must either be retrieved on one's own or one needs to rely on another individual or department to deliver the equipment. This adds additional work to either retrieve the equipment or schedule its delivery. Scheduling delivery ahead of time is particularly convenient for busy faculty members, although reliability of service is often problematic. Additional time and effort is then required to resolve the problem and obtain the equipment. Reserving equipment online through the school's Web site is one way to ease the burden involved with Internet use in the classroom. If the program is set up well, a written request can verify an order to increase the reliability of this mechanism. Arriving at class early to assemble equipment or to ensure that it has already been assembled can help to avoid lost class time related to delays.

SUMMARY

The classroom of the future is likely to be based even more on technology than it is today. Use of the Internet is one way to integrate technology into the classroom. Internet use in the classroom can be faculty centered or student centered. Faculty can use the Internet to enhance lecture materials, to demonstrate appropriate Web sites, or to critique information online. Student Internet-based assignments can be done off site or in the classroom with presentation to their peers. Benefits of Internet use in the traditional classroom include lively presentations, real evaluation of information, and opportunities for cooperative learning. Drawbacks include increased faculty time and work and the possibility of Web sites not functioning at the needed time.

WEB SITE RECAP

American Dietetics Association
http://www.eatright.org

Common Questions About Integrating the Internet into the Classroom
http://www.iloveteaching.com/Intenetclass/index.htm

Foodfit.com
http://www.foodfit.com

Internet Activities for Foreign Language Classes
http://members.aol.com/maestro12/web/wadir.html

Internet in the Classroom: First Steps
http://home.swbell.net/jraneri/Internetintheclassroom.htm

Using the Internet in the Classroom
http://mason.gmu.edu/~montecin/IDOweb-w.htm

Your Internet Guides: Internet Primer
http://www.thirteen.org/edonline/primer

REFERENCES

Collins, T., & Dewees, S. (2001). Challenge and promise: Technology in the class-room. [Online.] Available: *http://www.ext.msstate.edu/srdc/publications/millennium.htm*.

Holloway, N., Kripps, B., Koepke, K., & Skiba, D. J. (2000). Evaluating health care information on the Internet. In J. J. Fitzpatrick & K. S. Montgomery (Eds.), *Internet resources for nurses* (pp. 197–213). New York: Springer Publishing Co.

Montgomery, K. S. (2000). Nutrition. In J. J. Fitzpatrick & K. S. Montgomery (Eds.), *Internet resources for nurses* (pp. 117–122). New York: Springer Publishing Co.

Morin, K. H. (2001). Diet, nutrition, and weight loss. In J. J. Fitzpatrick, C. Romano, & R. Chasek (Eds.), *The nurses' guide to consumer health Web sites* (pp. 54–56). New York: Springer Publishing Co.

Poindexter, S., & Basu, S. C. (2000). Technology, teamwork, and teaching meet in the classroom. In *EDUCAUSE2000: Thinking it through. Proceedings and post-conference materials*. [Online.] Available: *http://www.educause.edu/conference/e2000/proceedings.html*.

Romano, C. A., Hinegardner, P. G., & Phyillaier, C. R. (2000). Some guidelines for browsing the Internet. In J. J. Fitzpatrick & K. S. Montgomery (Eds.), *Internet resources for nurses* (pp. xv–xvii). New York: Springer Publishing Co.

Chapter 16

Continuing Education

Julia W. Aucoin

L ocal access and time are two of the biggest barriers to participation in continuing education (Aucoin, 1998). Use of the Internet addresses both of these barriers. Access requires only hardware, software, and a modem, whereas time is totally in the control of the participant. Internet-based continuing education offers the ultimate in flexibility, allowing 24-hour access to a potential client base of 2.7 million nurses.

GENERAL PRINCIPLES FOR EVALUATING CONTINUING-EDUCATION OFFERINGS

Principles of good continuing education are applicable whether it is live, self-paced, or Internet-based. Well-planned continuing education is based on appropriate learner needs assessment. This information can be collected through sources such as focus groups, management reports, clinical observations, surveys, or industry trends. Learner objectives are developed to reflect desired outcomes of the offering. In clinical practice, objectives tend to be at the level of application and analysis rather than limited to knowledge and comprehension. Competency-based learning models often found in clinical practice address the realities of the care environment. Content is organized to support the stated learning objectives. Teaching strategies are selected based on content and objectives in order to assist the learner in achieving these objectives. When the Internet is chosen as the mode of delivery, the facilitator has greater opportunities for creativity than might be found with a live presentation. Digitized video and photos, group discussion via chat rooms and bulletin boards, application work through open access to course content, and accessing real-time information through links to live Web sites can all enhance the learning activities. Opportunities for evaluation are also expanded when Internet technology is used. Multiple attempts at quizzes with randomly assigned questions, discussion among the facilitator and colleagues, submission of essay, or leaving the computer to work with a preceptor and submitting successes and challenges afford the learner and faculty options for evaluation that are appropriate.

When assessing an Internet-based continuing-education activity, learners will want to evaluate each of these features to decide if they are appropriate to their needs. For example, a session on urinary catheterization could have the very simple objectives: "At the end of this activity the learner should be able to identify the reasons for catheterization, identify the steps to catheterization, and properly document the catheterization procedure." Or the objectives could be at a much higher level, for example: "At the end of this activity the learner should be able to teach self-catheterization techniques to patients, manage the patient with a difficult catheterization, and evaluate the effects of catheterization on the patient's other systems." The first set of objectives approximates what nursing students have to learn, and therefore does not provide much opportunity for growth or advancement. The second set of objectives is more advanced and would be more appropriate for the practicing nurse who is working with urologic patients. The question can then be posed, "Why are both levels of continuing education available on the Internet?" It is important to remember that anyone can place content on the Internet and these products will be at varying levels of quality. It is up to the consumer to shop wisely.

According to American Nurses Credentialing Center Commission on Accreditation's *Manual for Accreditation as a Provider of Continuing Nursing Education* (2001a), these key elements must be present in order to award continuing education credit:

- Continuing education activities are developed in response to, and with consideration for, the unique education needs of the organization's target audience
- Each education activity has an identified purpose and educational objective for the learner

- The education activity is planned by a Nurse Planner and others who have content expertise and represent the target audience
- Each education activity is congruent with its purpose and educational objectives
- Teaching/learning strategies are congruent with objectives and content
- Contact hours are determined in a logical and defensible manner, consistent with the objectives, content, teaching/learning strategies, and target audience
- There is a clearly defined method for evaluating the effectiveness of each continuing education activity, including learner input
- Revisions are made to ongoing continuing education activities based on evaluation data and participant input (ANCC, 2001a, p. 40).

The same criteria for educational design can be found in the companion manual for approvers (ANCC, 2001b). With these latest criteria, ANCC, the largest organization for accrediting continuing education activities in nursing, has broadened the opportunities for topics to be addressed in nursing continuing education. Therefore, opportunities will abound for development of new continuing education activities in communication and computer use, in addition to new clinical skills. At the same time, consumers must look carefully at the objectives before choosing and paying for an activity to ensure that the learning experience will meet their needs.

MODELS IN PRACTICE

Specialty Nursing Organization Resources

Many specialty organizations have begun to offer continuing education opportunities as part of their member benefits. In addition to publishing monographs and planning conferences, association leaders are directing their members to other strategies to meet their learning needs. The American Association of Critical Care Nurses (*www.aacn.org*) has several modules available online for improvements in the care of the critical-care patient, as does the Association for periOperative Registered Nurses (*www.aorn.org*) and the Association of Women's Health, Obstetrical, and Neonatal Nurses (*www.awhonn.org*).

Specialty nursing organizations have access to a plethora of clinical experts to develop quality continuing education. They often employ an educator who can guide the design process. Using their own resources or those of their management company, they can purchase or access a learning platform and server to support e-learning. These activities are generally available at a discount for members of the association.

For Profit

The Internet is a wonderful medium for the entrepreneur. Access to a domain name can be purchased for a mere $30 annual fee and Web design software is available at many office supply centers. If the company participates in the ANCC accreditation system, then there is an indication that planning follows the ANCC principles and thus there is an inherent degree of quality. As with attending a live presentation, the consumer should be able to judge the objectives, the faculty expertise, and the duration of the activity for appropriateness prior to purchase.

Publishing Companies

Several of the large publishers of nursing and health care texts and journals have moved into the electronic environment to provide continuing-education offerings. They are able to offer continuing-education components of their journal products through the Internet for a small fee. Publishers are able to increase their market penetration beyond the usual purchased subscriptions by offering continuing education. Often, portions of the activity are available free of charge to encourage participation.

Nursing students probably benefit the most from these sites, as they can download and print articles from the publisher's virtual library without stepping into a physical library. The student can read the article without needing to submit the continuing education quiz or the fee for credit.

University Continuing Education Departments

As universities use electronic environments to deliver their credit courses at a distance to graduate and undergraduate students, it becomes cost-effective and easy to use this learning platform to deliver continuing education to their alumni and the community. As the university already owns the server and may already have a supporting infrastructure, it is relatively easy for their teaching faculty to adapt some existing courses or lectures into Internet-based course work. What better way to share the expertise of faculty than to distribute his/her teachings via the Internet to a broader audience than could attend live classes.

Oftentimes the university continuing education department has developed a cooperative relationship with hospitals and other health care facilities to provide education that meets common needs. Using the Internet modality allows them to reach a broader audience.

STRENGTHS AND WEAKNESSES OF USING THE INTERNET IN CONTINUING EDUCATION

One must be very clear about the difference between a "page turner" and an online course. The Internet allows for the inclusion of both. However, a "page turner," one in which the individual reads text and then answers a brief quiz (as one would find in a journal), can be difficult to complete on the Internet, as reading lengthy text on a computer screen is fatiguing to the eyes. This mode of learning via the Internet has only one benefit: the journal doesn't have to be physically in front of you. A learning module can be widely accessible, printed locally, and the responses may require submissions via regular mail with a check, or possibly electronically if the site supports e-commerce.

In contrast, an online course offers both content and faculty-student interaction. The best courses also offer student-student interaction through the use of communication tools (e.g., bulletin board, chat, and e-mail). This interaction allows the student to validate learning, explore new information, and grow from the online experience. Content may be delivered via a textbook, Internet links, or even field experiences, yet its application is managed through course facilitation. In such courses students may feel more freedom to express their opinions, post their questions, and challenge the thinking of their peers.

Shopping on the Internet poses a problem for the consumer. When purchasing a sweater, there is a creatively worded description with a two-dimensional photo. It is not until the sweater is delivered that you can be sure of its texture and suitability. Consumer selection of continuing education on the Internet can also pose shopping challenges. The consumer must be knowledgeable of the characteristics of good quality products. Some companies provide "page turners" with content that is common to most nursing students, and may not have undergone any clinical or peer review. Yet, the best products could be overlooked due to their expense or the lack of a glitzy marketing campaign to attract the average nurse. See the resource list at the end of this chapter for recommendations.

PRACTICAL CONSIDERATIONS AND NECESSARY RESOURCES

In order to participate in Internet education, the learner must have hardware, software, and a modem sufficient to support the particular type of course. Particular course requirements will be found in the initial description of the course or course brochure, since many online courses are marketed through regular mail (Draves, 2000). Online courses are designed to be downloaded using a minimum 28.8 k modem. Faster speeds will lessen wait time. Learners can only tolerate about one hour of time at the computer, similar to the classroom. Breaking the content up into meaningful modules can help with comprehension and progression. Courses can be long, 24 contact hours for example, but should have an "activation" feature whereby the learner can stop and then resume the content without having to search for the previous stopping point. An orientation module may be necessary to familiarize the learner with how to use the technology prior to beginning the assignments.

HISTORICAL DEVELOPMENT OF INTERNET USE IN CONTINUING EDUCATION

The number of nurses annually who need continuing education changes from year to year. Reasons for this are related to each state's changing requirements for relicensure, and to nurses and nurse practitioners attaining certification or needing recertification. Thankfully, each year Yoder-Wise (2001) dedicates the editorial of the first issue of *The Journal of Continuing Education in Nursing* (*http://www. slackinc.com/allied/jcen/jcenhome.htm*) to an update of these requirements, providing continuing education institutions across the nation a current list of the amount and type of academic credit needed by their customers. In addition, mobile nurses have a greater need for independence from site-based learning. Many continuing education providers experience an increase in sales immediately before license renewal time.

Distance education has evolved over time. Armstrong, Gessner, and Cooper (2000) provide a chronology of distance education from mail order and radio delivery of courses, to teleconferencing and Internet use. As technology changes, so do the opportunities for delivery. As continuing education via the Internet is a consumer-based business, the decision to compete is based on how many nurses have access to computers and the Internet for home study. One must be careful to differentiate access to computers at the workplace from home access, because often the workplace computer is limited to work applications and does not afford the time to study that continuing education may require. The rise and fall of the dotcoms has affected Internet-based continuing education with several companies opening, closing, or merging in recent years.

FUTURE DIRECTIONS FOR FURTHER DEVELOPMENT

Faculty development in strategies for providing quality continuing education using technology is necessary for success. There are online and onsite courses to teach faculty these skills. It is equally important to know the audience and their learning needs, however. Today's new graduate is more comfortable with a computer and may already have had an online experience in school. Therefore, the numbers of nurses for whom Internet continuing education has appeal will increase. Nurses who have been in practice for some time may not be as comfortable with computers or Internet use, and may need additional assistance to complete Internet-based continuing education.

SUMMARY

As the Internet flourishes, so does its applications. Online education is one of the most exciting changes in teaching strategies. Access and time are the two biggest barriers to participation in continuing education via the Internet. Both of these barriers are in the control of the learner.

Continuing education offerings are available from a number of reputable sources. As with any fee-for-service activity, evaluation of quality is up to the learner.

RESOURCES

www.dollarceu.com—A company that offers continuing education for as little as $2.00 per activity, offering hundreds of topics

www.mylearningcommunity.org—A partnership between Cross Country University and Graphic Education Corporation

www.net-learning.com—A company that offers both JCAHO required topics and nursing continuing education

www.nursingceu.com—A nurse-owned company that offers many clinical topics ranging from quite simple to comprehensive and complex

http://nursing.iupui.edu/LifelongLearning—Provides nursing continuing education and training for faculty to learn how to provide online education

WEB SITE RECAP

American Association of Critical Care Nurses
http://www.aacn.org

Association for periOperative Registered Nurses
http://www.aorn.org

Association for Women's Health, Obstetrics, and Neonatal Nurses
http://www.awhonn.org

The Journal of Continuing Education in Nursing
http://www.slackinc.com/allied/jcen/jcenhome.htm

REFERENCES

American Nurses Credentialing Center. (2001a). *Manual for accreditation as a provider of continuing nursing education.* Washington, DC: Author.
American Nurses Credentialing Center. (2001b). *Manual for accreditation as an approver of continuing nursing education.* Washington, DC: Author.

Armstrong, M., Gessner, B., & Cooper, S. S. (2000). POTS, PANS, and PEARLs: The nursing profession's rich history with distance education for a new century of nursing. *The Journal of Continuing Education in Nursing, 31*, 63–70, 94–95.

Aucoin, J. (1998). Participation in continuing nursing education by staff development specialists. *Journal of Nursing Staff Development, 14,* 5.

Draves, W. (2000). *Teaching online.* River Falls, WI: LERN.

Yoder-Wise, P. (2001). State and certifying boards CE requirements. *Journal of Continuing Education in Nursing, 32,* 5–13.

Other Applications

Other Applications

Chapter 17

Health Care Policy and Legal Issues

Carole P. Jennings

I nformation and communication technologies have advanced health care professionals to a new age. The number of U.S. households with personal computers and access to the Internet has dramatically risen from 8% in 1984 to well over 60% today. Additionally, nearly every public library offers access to the Internet. The volume of information on the World Wide Web is so vast that even the best search engines have catalogued only about 28% of it (Eng et al., 1998).

Much of the information on the Internet is health related, in fact, researching health information is one of the most popular reasons for using the Internet. Today, the Internet possesses formidable power as consumers turn to the Web for health information to create their own custom venues for "virtual health care." This means access to health education and advice when they want it, where they want it, and from whom they want it.

Easy and increased access to health information on the Internet supports people in making informed health care decisions, promotes an empowered health care consumer, encourages the development of self-care strategies, provides access to emotional support from peers, and leads to improved health status by communicating the necessary components for a healthy lifestyle.

An important, yet rarely mentioned, side effect of the health information revolution is the decentralization and democratization of knowledge traditionally held by the medical experts (Eng et al., 1998). The so-called, "medical mystique" is fast eroding as patients "surf the net" and often outpace their provider's knowledge of the latest scientific research, clinical trial, or treatment protocol. The same can be said for health policy and legal information. In the past, policy elites and legal experts made the complex, difficult interpretations in public policy debates and legal arenas. They then conveyed their expert judgments to the public. Today, it is often the ordinary layperson who turns the tide in policy decision-making, harnessing the powerful tools of information technology to access the same information resources used by policy and legal gurus. Consumers are increasingly taking ownership of information about health care and that fact alone is dramatically changing the way health care and legal policy decisions are made.

Milstead (1999) proposed that nurses can stand tall in their multiple roles of provider of care, educator, administrator, political activist, consultant, and policy-maker. Unfortunately, the roles of political activist and policy-maker have been given short shrift by nurses who do not see these skills as central to their practice of nursing. The author adds that if nurses do not exercise their roles as political activists and policy-makers, their professional power base and influence on our nation's health will greatly diminish.

This chapter facilitates nurses' involvement in the political, policy, and legal aspects of health care. The policy process is used as an organizing framework for considering how nurses can access information and participate in policy development. The policy process is dynamic and fluid, and its very nature underscores the tremendous advantage of information technology as a tool to help nurses easily access data and use it to build their case for action to public officials. The chapter introduces the reader to examples of key health policy and legal Internet sites, provides criteria for evaluating information sources on the Internet, and presents a brief overview of policy and legal issues that are part and parcel of information technology.

THE POLICY PROCESS

The policy process is a sequential process much like the basic problem-solving process used by nurses to accomplish patient care planning. Policy formulation occurs in a number of ways: the enactment of legislation and its accompanying rules and regulations, which have the weight of law, administrative decisions in institutions, and judicial decisions that interpret the law (Hanley, 1998). Public policy encompasses anything a government chooses to do or not do. Health policy is a purposeful course of action to deal with the health issues confronting a society. Health policies in place today guide the operation of the Medicare and Medicaid programs, set medical privacy standards, and structure the operation of the Children's Health Insurance Program (CHIP) and rural health clinics.

Politics is increasingly intertwined with public policy-making, which is defined as "the allocation of scarce resources." Special interest groups lobby the Congress and the executive branch to gain access to scarce health care dollars and resources. They are often characterized as policy stakeholders. A policy stakeholder includes elected or appointed officials, interest group representatives, and individuals who are directly involved in shaping a particular policy and who may be affected directly by the policy outcome or the impact of its implementation (Hanley, 1998). It takes a tremendous act of political will to make major health policy decisions/changes as seen in the recent debate about patients' bill of rights legislation in the U.S. Congress.

The policy process refers to the steps a proposal moves through from conceptualization to a fully operational program. The four stages of the process include: (1) policy agenda setting; (2) policy formulation; (3) policy implementation; and (4) policy evaluation. Each stage of the process is subject to influence by informed nurses who are knowledgeable about the process and know how and when to intervene. It is important to know how to obtain information on health care or legal issues at each stage of the process, and information technology is a tool that allows anyone to obtain needed information by simply sitting at their personal computer and clicking on the appropriate Web site. The policy process is very dynamic in nature, and the stages are open to multiple feedback loops and influences, particularly the power of the informed public and special interest group advocates.

Stage 1: Policy Agenda Setting

The first step in setting a policy agenda is identification of a policy problem, a situation that produces needs or dissatisfaction for which relief is sought (Hanley, 1998). Only those public problems that finally reach a policy makers' attention qualify as a policy problem. A legitimate policy problem initiates the policy process. The confluence of problems, proposed solutions, and political circumstances that make the time "ripe for action" lead to the development of legislation. Nurses can participate in this stage of the process by raising issues of concern, bringing the issue to the public's attention, networking and forming coalitions with other interested parties, and formulating an action plan to resolve the problem. The goal is to magnify one's power base so that official policy-makers take note and take action. Nurses can use the media, letters to the editor, spots on television and radio talk shows, speaking at public gatherings (town meetings), writing for organization newsletters, contacting members of Congress or the state legislature, and publishing research findings to get the word out about the health problem. Setting up a Web site to provide information about the problem to the public is an excellent approach, as well as participating in a list serv or chat room to promote dialogue about the issue with interested professional colleagues or community leaders and activists. Web sites for the American Nurses Association, *http://www.ana.org* and the American Academy of Nurse Practitioners, *http://www.aanp.org* are two examples of organizational sites that provide policy and political information and alerts for nurses.

Stage 2: Policy Formulation

At this stage, policy options are considered and proposals are actually formulated, put into legislative language, and introduced into the legislative body. Often hearings are held and expert witnesses are invited to give testimony presenting their perspective on the policy issue or problem. This is a very technical phase of the policy process during which information is collected, analyzed, and disseminated to the press, to the public, and to other policy-makers. It is also the stage that is open and permeable to outside influence. Nurses must become adept at going to Web sites, "calling up" bills of interest, and responding to policy-makers. Once the site appears, the nurse can enter a topic area such as domestic violence or a bill number and then download the entire piece of legislation. Often, e-mailing the sponsors of the legislation or setting up an appointment directly with the policy-maker or his/her legislative aide can be an effective response to the legislation.

Compromise and negotiation are the soul of politics and it is here, at the policy formulation phase, that strategies to promote them are most crucial. Legislative proposals that are deemed worthy of action are introduced, referred to the committee or committees of jurisdiction, marked-up, passed out of committee, and taken to the floor of the chamber of Congress considering the legislation. The same process is repeated in the other chamber. This process is almost always a lengthy one and provides ample opportunity for intervention and influence. Legislative bodies must begin to hear more from informed professional nurses. Web sites to reach the U.S. House of Representatives, the Senate, *The Congressional Record*, and *The Washington Post* are as follows: The U.S. Congress: *http://www.congress.gov*, Congressional Record Text: *http://thomas.loc.gov*, and *The Washington Post: http://www.washingtonpost.com*. Additionally, each legislator has his or her own Web site and e-mail address so quick access to the policymaker is possible.

Stage Three: Policy Implementation

This is the phase of the policy process when regulations are written by executive branch agencies and authorizing policies are transformed into workable programs. In the implementation phase, much of the responsibility for policymaking shifts from the legislative branch to the executive branch of government. Executive branch agencies like the Department of Health and Human Services and the Justice Department primarily exist to implement the policies mandated by legislation. Nurses can monitor *The Federal Register* and corresponding state publications for notices of proposed rulemaking and the publication of final rules and regulations, and they can also respond to proposed rules during the public comment period. At this phase it is important to be watchful, ensuring that the legislative intent is fully reflected in the rulemaking process. Proposed and final rules can be accessed from the *Federal Register* Web site: *http://www.access.gpo.gov/su_docs/aces/aces140.html*

Longest (1994) wrote that "although the executive branch bears most of the responsibility for implementing policies, the legislative branch maintains an oversight responsibility and often a continuing re-authorization and annual appropriations responsibility. There is also a judicial dimension to the implementation phase: administrative law judges hear the appeals of the people or organizations that are dissatisfied with the way implementation of policies impacts on them" (pp. 83–84). Legislation, as well as subsequent regulations, can be challenged in the courts. This aspect of the policymaking process attests to the delicate system of checks and balances set forth in the Constitution in 1789. That document laid out our structure of government and allocated powers to each of the three branches: legislative, executive, and judicial.

Stage Four: Policy Evaluation

Any policy evaluation process must ask, "Did the policy work?" Additionally, it is important to query, "Whom did the program in question help and whom did it harm?" This stage is often referred to as the forgotten stage of the policy process. The U.S. General Accounting Office (GAO) and the Agency for Healthcare Research and Quality (AHRQ) (clinical outcomes research agency) are two government agencies that are charged with the task of evaluating public policy. Nurses can be instrumental in bringing attention to available reports that evaluate existing policy. They may also encourage, promote, and initiate the evaluation of existing health and legal policy. Their respective Web sites are: U.S. General Accounting Office (GAO), *http://www.gao.gov* and Agency for Healthcare Research and Quality, *http://www.ahrq.gov.*

This phase has also been called the policy modification phase because the operational experiences gained in implementing policies, and the outcomes, perceptions, and consequences of implementation often trigger future policy formulation and implementation (Longest, 1994).

Other important Web sites in the health policy and legal arenas for nurses include: the state and federal supreme court and the networks of federal and state courts; one's state legislature, legislators, and the governor's office; the national state boards of nursing and a nurse's individual state board of nursing. The last site can alert the practicing nurse to changes in the Nurse Practice Act in his or her state, such as the posting of declaratory rulings, which may expand the nursing activities included within a nurse's scope of practice.

EVALUATING INTERNET RESOURCES

Even though the Internet can provide unlimited access to health policy and legal information, there is no guarantee that the information is accurate, credible, or reliable. The Internet is open to all, and anyone can create a Web site and post information. The user of information technology must be vigilant and able to evaluate the information as well as the source that produced it. Milstead (1999) presented the following evaluation guidelines: (a) Look at the *author*—is he or she named along with credentials, professional reputation, and affiliation? There may even be a link to the author's curriculum vitae to assess credentials. (b) What information is available about the *type of site*?— Look at the URL to see what type of site is represented. Is it an educational institution (edu), a company (com), an organizational site (org), or a government site (gov)? The URL designation generally tells the nurse who is sponsoring the site and one can then determine if any overview process exists to ensure the accuracy of information. (c) What about the *timeliness* of the information presented—is it old news and outdated information? If the site uses a search engine to update information, one may find a date in the search engine results. The date indicated is the last time the information was updated. (d) The *content* may be based on fact or opinion. Is the content clear, easy to understand, and accurate? Does it contain any bias? Is the information consistent with other sources that are considered credible (Nelson, 1999)? If these guidelines are followed, the nurse can be more confident in using the information obtained from the Internet to define a health policy problem, develop an action plan for solving the problem, implement the plan, and evaluate the results. Information technology helps the nurse to fully participate in the policy process. The following sites are good sources for evaluation criteria and tools that help the nurse distinguish quality information from misinformation: *http://www.ciolek. com/WWWVL-InfoQuality.html, http://www2.widener.edu/Wolfgram-Memorial-Library/pyramid.htm, http://library.albany.edu/Internet/evaluate. html* (Nelson, 1999, p. 273).

DEVELOPMENT OF INFORMATION TECHNOLOGY

Some of the current policy and legal issues that impact the development of information technology are:

- Confidentiality of patient information—how does one build in privacy protections?
- Licensure of providers—how can policy best address licensing practitioners who practice routinely across state jurisdictional lines,

and who is liable and who will prosecute in malpractice cases? This is of particular concern in the use of telehealth technology.
- Issues surrounding public and private reimbursement and subsidization of information sources.
- Antitrust behaviors—who will control the flow and use of information on the Internet? Will we see a dramatic increase in monopolistic market behavior?
- Fraud and abuse—what protections, such as whistle-blower protections, are in place to prevent these behaviors?
- Telecommunication contracting—who owns the rights?
- Development of ethical standards to guide production and use of information on the Internet.

SUMMARY

Goldsmith (2000) described how the Internet has exploded during the late 1990s into a powerful new social institution. He continues, "the Internet is only incidentally a broadcast medium. Rather, it is more like a flexible and powerful new nervous system for the economy and society" (p. 148). The challenge of the next decades will be transforming information into knowledge, dealing with the decay rate of scientific knowledge (particularly a problem for educational settings and institutions, and practicing health care professionals), and working with and caring for the cyber-assisted patient (Goldsmith, 2000).

Health information technology is changing the way nurses can participate in public policy as well. Access to the latest and the best information about health care trends, statistics, and discussions among policy and legal experts, opens the world of decision-making in these important areas to the individual nurse and to nursing organizations. Knowledge and information is indeed power. Nurses must harness this power to promote the needs of health care consumers and the survival of nursing itself as a professional enterprise. Part of the new role of nurses as political activists is policy and legal advocacy. Nurses must be active and assertive in the policy arena to truly meet the needs of patients, families, and communities. Thanks to information technology, the nurses of tomorrow can be key players in every public policy debate.

WEB SITE RECAP

A Modular Approach to Teaching/Learning the World Wide Web
http://www2.widener.edu/Wolfgram-Memorial-Library/pyramid.htm

Agency for Healthcare Research and Quality
http://www.ahrq.gov

American Academy of Nurse Practitioners
http://www.aanp.org

American Nurses Association
http://www.ana.org

Congressional Record Text
http://thomas.loc.gov/

Federal Register
http://www.access.gpo.gov/su_docs/aces/aces140.html

Information Quality World Wide Web Virtual Library
http://www.ciolek.com/WWWVL-InfoQuality.html

The U.S. Congress
http://www.congress.gov

The Washington Post
http://www.washingtonpost.com

U.S. General Accounting Office (GAO)
http://www.gao.gov

University at Albany Libraries Evaluating Internet Resources
http://library.albany.edu/Internet/evaluate.html

REFERENCES

Eng, T., Maxfield, A., Patrick, K., Deering, M. J., Ratzan, S., & Gustafon, D. (1998). Policy perspectives: Access to health information and support: A public highway or a private road? *Journal of the American Medical Association, 280*, 1371–1375.

Goldsmith, J. (2000). How will the Internet change our health system? *Health Affairs, 19*(1), 148–156.

Hanley, B. (1998). Policy development and analysis. In D. Mason & J. Leavitt (Eds.), *Policy and politics in nursing and health care* (3rd ed., pp. 125–138). Philadelphia: W. B. Saunders.

Longest, B. (1994). *Health policymaking in the United States.* Ann Arbor, MI: AUPHA Press/Health Administration Press.

Milstead, J. A. (1999). *Health policy and politics: A nurse's guide.* Gaithersburg, MD: Aspen.

Nelson, R. (1999). The Internet and health care policy information. In J. A. Milstead (Ed.), *Health policy and politics: A nurse's guide* (pp. 257–276). Gaithersburg, MD: Aspen.

_____ Chapter **18**

The Research Setting

Jan V. R. Belcher and Carol Holdcraft

T|he Internet was originally conceived and sponsored by the National Science Foundation (NSF) as a way to connect researchers at several national supercomputing centers so that they could share ideas (Wheeler & O'Kelly, 1999). The National Science Foundation Network (NFSNET) backbone became so popular with commercial traffic that a private network was established; this network grew into the current Internet system. With this background, it is easy to see that the Internet is a fertile setting for research activity for many scholars who seek communication with peers as well as access to potential research subjects. This chapter will discuss the use of the Internet as a communication medium among nurse researchers, their clinical nursing colleagues, and the clients and public they serve.

The Internet has made the nursing community a global village with expanding opportunities to discover and share information. Collaboration and consultation with nurse experts as well as dissemination of research findings is becoming more rapid and convenient for more nurses than ever before. The Internet provides access to health statistics and research instruments, as well as potential research subjects. Survey research, in particular, has found a niche on the Internet, although it has some notable pitfalls. Nurses have been innovators in using the capabilities of the Internet in research, and as the medium expands and technologies advance, the potential use of the Internet as a research tool is enormous.

INTERNET COMMUNICATION

The Internet has already greatly enhanced communication about research among nurses. Electronic mail (e-mail) has been the major vehicle for this enhanced communication. The nurse in the office, at home, or even in the car, can quickly e-mail a researcher to ask a question clarifying a method or about a point made in a published article. Often the researcher responds to a question within 24 hours, thus shortening correspondence time by several days. The nurse and the researcher can even be located in different countries and correspond within minutes using e-mail.

Research tools have become more available with Internet access. Nurses can search the Internet for a research topic using a search engine, and then go to a specific research center's or individual researcher's Web page. From the Web page, the nurse can examine the research tool and then e-mail the author asking permission to use the tool. Several times researchers have received e-mail questions asking which tools are available in a specific research area. Many Web sites have distributed research tools. For example, the Centers for Disease Control and Prevention, the World Health Organization, and other private vendors have distributed the majority of the 145,000 copies of Epi Info and Epi Map, computer software programs for epidemiology and research, through the Internet (Harbage & Dean, 1999). This accessibility enormously decreases the amount of time it takes for a nurse to locate and use the research tool.

Research bulletin boards and listervs are becoming important vehicles for research dialogue. Electronic bulletin boards are used to post messages and transmit information that is shared with all users. A listserv is an e-mail subscription list that distributes all e-mail messages to all subscribers. Individual researchers or professional research organizations can use bulletin boards and listservs to communicate news items or specific information.

Besides e-mail and bulletin boards, video broadcasts have also become an important medium for communication. Video broadcasts allow for real-time video and audio recording and distribution over the Internet. This medium allows for different professionals in different geographical locations to view the video simultaneously. Clinicians and researchers could have global research conferences to discuss a research protocol or expedite dissemination of research. Video broadcasts also allow for Web site storage of the video so that researchers can view the video at another time from the Web site. Video broadcasts allow nurses and researchers to view the same research information or clinical situations simultaneously, or at different times. At the present time, video broadcasts are expensive for many organizations and the quality of the broadcasts can vary, but this will become a major medium of communication in the future.

In their study on video broadcasts, Levy, Lash, Iverson, and Dixon (2000) used a live-stream video broadcast over the Internet to present a medical and rehabilitation conference on a rare disease, fibrodysplasia ossifcans progressiva. The Web site was accessed 83 times in two days including two sites in The Netherlands and Israel. Levy and colleagues (2000) concluded that the Internet was a viable tool for communication. They stated that the cost of the video broadcast was reasonable, with $2,000–$4,000 in 1998 computer requirements and an additional 5 hours of training for a computer-literate individual to record and broadcast.

COLLABORATION AND CONSULTATION

The Internet has greatly enhanced collaboration and consultation among researchers. Through e-mail and Web pages, researchers all over the world can be contacted. Researchers can be on different continents and have daily contact with each other. This collaboration is critical in multisite studies or when external consultation is needed quickly. In addition, an expert researcher can work on several projects simultaneously which saves time and is more cost effective than traveling or telephoning from one geographical site to another.

With the Internet, the research team can have more diverse members. Not all members need to be in the same location. Nurses can therefore incorporate other disciplines of research and other clinicians from all over the world into the research team. This accessibility will produce quality research with diverse views and applications.

One way that access to research data can be streamlined is by the creation of intranets. Intranets are private networks that use Internet technologies (Gillespie, 2000). Intranets are created by organizations for communication among employees in different locations within the organization. The goal of intranets is to create easy-to-navigate communication devoted exclusively to the business of the organization. Intranets can be used to facilitate communication among the research team. Besides sending direct e-mail to research project team members, research reports can be posted on the intranet so all team members can use the information simultaneously. The intranet has the promise of creating an efficient communication infrastructure for the research team. Intranets have also been used to conduct clinical trials (Kelley, 2000). Some computer software packages such as Microsoft Project allow for creating project Web sites for research team use.

One concern of creating an intranet where employees can access organizational information from home or other work locations is information security. In further developing intranets, security must be a very high priority (Gillespie, 2000). Using the intranet, the research data collector could download data on a laptop computer from a different geographical clinical site directly into the intranet databases through portals for easy accessibility and analysis. The researcher needs to ensure that the data is secure and not available for others to view.

RESEARCH DISSEMINATION

Through the Internet, nurses are accessing research with only a click of the mouse. This is exciting because the Internet has the potential of disseminating research quickly to many clinically practicing nurses. Nurses cannot only search research databases, but they can also scan research abstracts. On the Internet, the number of full-text research articles is growing, and many professional journals such as the *Online Journal of Issues of Nursing, Nursing Research, American Journal of Nursing,* and *British Medical Journal* are posted on the Internet. At this time, several journals are free to users, but many have subscription fees. This technology not only allows for quick access, but also a shorter time between completed research and research being applied into practice. The publication lag time can be greatly decreased. In addition, communication time between publisher and author is condensed. For example, one author submitted an article directly to the editor of a professional journal to be published via e-mail. Within a week, the editor had responded via e-mail with written comments on the article to be revised for publication. This same process, without e-mail, could take several weeks or months.

Databases for research articles have become commonplace and are still growing. Some research databases on the Web require a member subscription, whereas others are free. Some research is accessible through governmental Web sites, and others are made accessible by organizations or individuals. Two of the most common databases are PubMed (*http://www.nim.nih.gov*) and CINAHL (*http://www.cinahl.com*). These databases are discussed in more detail in chapters 5 and 13.

Because there are a variety of sources for research dissemination, the nurse must carefully scrutinize the source of the information to determine its quality. Web authors are often skilled at presenting research findings with biases for selling products or giving misinformation. Sometimes research findings are condensed so that the nurse does not receive adequate information to evaluate the research her/himself. Wolfgram Memorial Library (1999) created a checklist to evaluate Web-based information that includes authority, accuracy, objectivity, currency, and coverage. This checklist would also be useful to the nurse to determine the quality of the source of the research findings.

Another disadvantage to this explosion of fingertip Internet information is that many times, clinical nurses and nursing students are using only the Internet to find research information. Although the Internet is rapidly expanding, it still does not have the comprehensive resources that the library does. At this time, not all the library resources are on the Internet. In addition, although the Internet may be easily accessed at home or work, many research articles are condensed or rewritten with a bias to support a Web author's position. Devlin and Burke (1997) asserted that although the Internet might be considered the ultimate reference tool, it provides no assurance of quality information.

Another caution with using the Internet for examining current research is the problem with Web site consistency. Belcher and Holdcraft (2000) found that only 80% of Web sites addressing depression were consistently available over a three-month period. At this time, the Internet has a phenomenon of vanishing Web sites and information. Web authors deleting or changing Web page information, and technology problems making Web sites unavailable to users, cause vanishing Web sites. Consistent documentation of the source of information is many times very difficult to find. Nurses should be aware of this phenomenon. Web page information can be printed from Web sites and the Web site can be bookmarked for further evaluation of its consistency.

Nurses can also use the Internet to disseminate research to the public. Approximately half of United States users searched the Internet for health information (Eng et al., 1998). Since the public is increasingly using the Internet to manage their health, nurses could use this medium for disseminating research to the public. Nurse researchers have been criticized for not making their research readily available to the public in easy, understandable language. Nursing Web sites that are easy to locate and navigate could also present research findings and applications to targeted groups in the public such as research on cardiac, depression, or diabetes health management issues.

CONDUCTING SURVEY RESEARCH

The Internet provides a new medium for researchers to access a global subject pool, and would seem to be an ideal method for conducting survey research. The ability to draw on subjects from far away is a definite advantage for researchers using the Internet. Other advantages include lower costs for mailing and coding, shorter turnaround time, access to hard-to-reach or rare samples, and fewer coding errors than with conventional surveys (Zhang, 1999).

However, some pitfalls and disadvantages have been determined by researchers attempting to use this new medium for their research. The current online population is not representative of the general public. Those with access to the Internet are inherently different from those without access, as has been noted by authors who study the "digital divide" (National Telecommunications and Information Administration, October 2000). There are differences among the connected and the unconnected with regard to racial groups, age, income levels, educational levels, and geographic regions. A potential for biased samples and biased returns exists due to unequal access to the Internet, lack of comfort with Internet survey formats, self-selection bias, unintended respondents, and multiple responses from the same person (Zhang, 1999). Researchers must take into account these potential biases when conducting survey research on the Internet.

In an attempt to determine how patients who participate in an online survey might differ from patients located for a study through conventional means, researchers compared these two subject pools (Soetikno, Mrad, Pao, & Lenert, 1997). They found ulcerative colitis patients who responded to the Internet survey were younger and more symptomatic, as measured by their responses to the illness questionnaire (Soetikno, Mrad, Pao, & Lenert, 1997). In another survey researchers gave respondents who had difficulty completing an online survey the option to print and send by facsimile (fax) their responses. They found that respondents who were more comfortable with computers tended to be more successful in completing the Web-based survey (Schleyer & Forrest, 2000). Zhang (1999) found that respondents who chose the Web for response had higher perceived ability to use the Internet, used the Web more frequently, and were younger than respondents who chose to mail or fax their responses.

Survey forms can be designed for online use to improve the accuracy and completeness of responses. Respondents come with a wide variety of backgrounds and there is a discrepancy in their sophistication in computer usage. Therefore the forms need very clear directions. Survey questions should be placed on sequential screens rather than one long page. Minimal need to scroll helps assure that all parts will be read. Response forms can use list boxes, radio buttons, check boxes, or circles to record answers to closed-ended questions. Open-ended questions can be answered via text fields. The form can be programmed to prevent multiple responses and to cue respondents to fill in missing responses before allowing them to proceed. However, sometimes respondents do not answer certain items by choice, or because the item does not apply to them, so care must be taken to allow for all possible appropriate responses. Several sources are published with guidelines for creating online survey instruments (Turner & Turner, 1999).

In addition to the time it normally takes to develop the content of a typical survey, time must be allocated to program the format of the survey for Internet usage. Pilot testing is an important step and should be done using typical respondents having a variety of Internet browsers, operating systems, Internet access providers, and modem speeds. Care must be taken that the responses be accurately coded into the data collection or scoring format. Early responses should be scrutinized for possible coding errors and corrections made rapidly. Although advanced programming features such as graphics and colors may make the survey instrument more appealing, the wide variety of computer equipment of respondents means it is better to keep the survey simple in design to keep the files small and easy to download.

When sampling bias and selection bias is of limited importance to the purpose of the research, samples can be recruited by targeting bulletin boards and search engines. Samples may be generated via e-mailed invitations to listservs. Some surveys are distributed by e-mail with respondents sending their completed survey back to the researcher via e-mail, fax, or conventional mail. One advantage of a Web-based survey over an e-mailed survey is greater anonymity for respondents (Lakeman, 1997; Zhang, 1999). As with the more typical paper-and-pencil surveys, incentives to completing the survey may be offered. Subjects with rare or hard to access conditions may be more readily recruited through Web sites that are directed toward providing information and support for these patients.

Passive net sampling is a method of sampling where researchers place a large number of catchwords related to the study in the "meta" section of the HTML code. These catchwords are designed to be used as index words by search engines. This method draws interested Web searchers to the site where they can be invited to participate in the Web survey (Senior, Phillips, Barnes, & David, 1999).

In general, the costs associated with doing a mailed survey increase with the number accessed. However, with online surveys, there is a breakeven point where the online version will be more economical since the cost is independent of the sample size. In one comparison, 275 was the breakeven point where the online version became cheaper (Schleyer & Forrest, 2000). Using another technique to save costs, qualitative data can be imported directly into qualitative analysis software without the expense of transcription.

ACCESS TO HEALTH STATISTICS AND DATA MINING

The Internet provides convenient access to numerous health statistics via government and health organization Web sites. The World Health Organization's Web site, (*www.who.org*), provides links to outbreaks of infectious diseases that are updated frequently with the most recent statistics. The National Center for Health Statistics (NCHS), which is part of the Centers for Disease Control and Prevention (CDC) (*http://www.cdc.gov*), has links to a data warehouse. This site has public-use downloadable files that are maintained on the CDC FTP file server. Data sets, documentation, and questionnaires from NCHS surveys are available. Some examples of survey data that are available include the National Health and Nutrition Examination Survey (NHANES), the National Health Care Survey (NHCS), and the National Health Interview Survey (NHIS). Tools such as the Statistical Export and Tabulation System (SETS) are available for researchers. This downloadable program gives data users the tools to access and manipulate large data sets on their personal computers. Graduate students and other researchers can use these data sets to perform statistical analyses to answer health relationship questions without having to go to the time and expense of collecting the primary data themselves.

Because many large health care databases are being created with the advent of the Internet and other technology, a new research method has been created—data mining. Data mining is the extraction of patterns and relationships hidden in the data within the databases (Abbott, 2000; Axer, Jantzen, & von Keyserlingk, 2000). Interdisciplinary research teams are becoming more involved in data mining. In Europe, a research team (Axer, Jantzen, & von Keyserlingk, 2000) developed Web-based software to mine data from an aphasic patient database. Their model produced 92% correct diagnoses supporting the idea that data mining can be clinically useful.

SUMMARY OF CURRENT RESEARCH

Nurses can use the Internet as a tool in the research process to find resources, collect data, and disseminate research. Most of the interdisciplinary research on the Internet has examined this area. In this summary of current research, Internet research is categorized into survey studies, descriptive studies of the Internet, and Internet intervention studies.

Survey Studies

The first category of Internet research is survey studies. Using the Internet for data collection in survey research has been a growing area of research. Thomas, Stamler, Lafreniere, and Dumala (2000), for example, found the Internet to be an effective tool when they studied an international sample of 593 women and their perception of breast health education and screening. Crownover (1998) used the Internet to survey patients with diabetes.

Another survey studied health care professionals, primarily nurses, in home health and hospice. Long, Greenberg, Isemurt, and Smith (2000) examined the use of the Internet and computers through a Web survey. Their sample was composed of 122 health care professionals in 38 states. They found that respondents used the Internet for various reasons including medical and disease information, product and service information, patient education, research, governmental information, education, accreditation information, and insurance information. The following personnel used the Internet in descending order: managers (91%), financial personnel (64%), educators (57%), quality management (56%), and nursing staff (32%). In this study, survey respondents wanted more Web-based instruction and computer assisted instruction that could be cost effective for home health and hospice organizations.

Descriptive Studies of the Internet

The second category of research includes descriptive research of the Internet. Nurses, along with other professionals, are beginning to study the quality of information posted on the Internet and its effect on the individual seeking the information, whether it is professionals, patients, or the general public. Researchers studying the Internet have unique challenges because the structure of the Internet is confusing and constantly changing (Belcher & Holdcraft, 2000).

Many descriptive studies focus on specific health problems. Diering and Palmer (2001) evaluated 265 Web sites for information about urinary incontinence. They found that most information was accurate, but critical analysis skills were needed to evaluate the posted information. Beredjklian, Bozentka, Steinberg, and Bernstein (2000) examined 250 Web sites for information on carpal tunnel syndrome. They found the information to be limited and of poor quality. Griffiths and Christensen (2000) evaluated 21 Web sites for depression information. They rated the sites as having poor quality. Belcher and Holdcraft (2000) evaluated 86 depression Web sites and found a variety of authors who publish Web sites with some information that could be harmful to the public. Suarez-Almazor, Kendall, and Dorgan (2001) evaluated 388 Web sites for arthritis information and found many sites to be for-profit companies advertising products. (For more information on evaluating Web sites, please see Holloway, Kripps, Koepke, and Skiba [2000] and Fitzpatrick, Romano, and Chasek [2001].)

In psychology, researchers are beginning to establish the Internet as a valid research medium (Smith & Senior, 2001). Krantz, Ballard, and Scher (1997) compared Internet and nonInternet responses regarding female body images and found no differences between groups. Another Internet study (Smith and Leigh, 1997) replicated a "pen and paper" study about fantasies and found comparable responses in the two studies.

Instead of Internet surveys, Rettie (2001) used focus groups to facilitate discussion of 32 participants' experience on the Internet. She applied the concept of flow to the Internet and consumer behavior. Internet information flow was defined as people being very absorbed in an activity such as surfing the Internet. In this study, approximately half of the participants experienced information flow while on the Internet. Factors that inhibited Internet flow included slow downloading time, poor site navigation, long registration forms, and irrelevant links. Factors that enhanced flow (e.g., quick downloading times, easy navigation, and short registration forms) promoted user interactivity and control.

Internet Intervention Studies

A third category of research, intervention studies, is in its infancy. Researchers are beginning to create and evaluate use of the Internet as an intervention strategy. Such strategies could include interactive Web sites, bulletin boards, e-mail, health and disease information, decision support, and/or Internet videoconferencing.

One intervention study used the Internet to create a system of computer technical support in private homes. Brennan, Moore, and Symth (1995) designed ComputerLink for Alzheimer's patient caregivers. ComputerLink was composed of an electronic bulletin board, disease information, and decision support. In a randomized clinical trial, the researchers found that the computer system was a feasible way to deliver services to Alzheimer's caregivers. In particular, asynchronous communication, communication that does not require that the caregivers be online at the same time, was important.

Another study examined the effect of computers in the home with persons living with AIDS. Flatley-Brennan (1998) studied whether a home-based computer network could reduce social isolation, and offer information and decision making assistance to persons living with AIDS. In a 6-month randomized trial, 31 people were in the experimental group. The researcher concluded that computer networks showed great promise in providing health services to homebound individuals. The experimental group was not resistant to learning the technology needed for the study. The communication system that consisted of e-mail, a public bulletin board, and an anonymous question and answer section was frequently used.

Web pages on the Internet were found to be a useful educational multimedia tool. Kim, Kim, and Kim (2001) created a breast self-examination program on the Internet using graphics, sound, text, and a social network through consultation in Korea. The sample consisted of 82 female volunteer university students. The researchers found that participants needed breast self-examination information and that patients would access this content via Web pages.

In one intervention study, the Internet was used to create a research network. Lau and Haywood (2000) used an interactive Web site and online surveys to create a virtual network that facilitated research utilization in community health. Over a two-year period, 25 health professionals from 17 health regions in Canada participated in a community health research program. This program addressed research methods, data analysis, computers, management, and health policy. This study described a conceptual model and processes that facilitated creating virtual networks to utilize technology to enhance work practices and incorporate research into clinical decision-making.

Another intervention study demonstrated higher-quality care and lower costs than in a standard neonatal intensive care unit (NICU). Gray and colleagues (2000) examined the impact of an Internet-based telemedicine program that provided medical, emotional, and informational support to parents of very-low-birth-weight infants during and after their NICU stay. After infants were randomized, the families in the experimental group were given home computers with an Internet browser and videoconferencing equipment. The control group was given standard NICU care. The 26 families who were in the experimental group reported an overall higher quality of care and earlier home discharge than the control group.

SUMMARY

In summary, the Internet is revolutionizing how nurses and the public receive information. Nurses are increasingly using the Internet for research and practice information. In the area of research, nurses can access Web sites for research article searches, abstract summaries, and even some full-text articles. The Internet allows for communication with experts and other colleagues and is becoming a valid research medium. Existing research methods can be adapted for use on the Internet along with the creation of new research methods. This medium is exploding and will provide nurses with even more data, information, experts, intervention strategies, and global access in the future.

WEB SITE RECAP

Centers for Disease Control
http://www.cdc.gov

World Health Organization
http://www.who.org

REFERENCES

Abbott, P. (2000). Knowledge discovery in large data sets: A primer for data mining application in health care. In Ball, Hannah, Newbold, & Douglas (Eds.), *Nursing informatics: Where caring and technology meet* (3rd ed.). New York: Springer-Verlag.

Axer, H., Jantzen, J., & von Keyserlingk, D. G. (2000). An aphasia database on the Internet: A model for computer-assisted analysis in aphasiology. *Brain and Language, 75*, 390–398.

Belcher, J. V., & Holdcraft, C. (2000). Discovering the mosaic of knowledge, hope and peril on the Web: A descriptive study of depression resources [Abstract]. *Proceedings of the 10th Annual Summer Institute in Nursing Informatics*, University of Maryland.

Beredjklian, P. K., Bozentka, D. J., Steinberg, D. R., & Bernstein, J. (2000). Evaluating the source and content of orthopaedic information on the Internet. *The Journal of Bone and Joint Surgery, 82A*, 1540–1543.

Brennan, P., Moore, S., & Smyth, K. (1995). The effects of a special computer network on care givers of persons with Alzheimer's disease. *Nursing Research, 44*, 166–172.

Crownover, A. J. (1998). Using the Internet to survey patients with diabetes [Abstract]. *Image: Journal of Nursing Scholarship, 30*, 392–393.

Devlin, B., & Burke, M. (1997). Internet: The ultimate reference tool? *Internet Research: Electronic Networking, Application and Policy, 7*(2), 101–108.

Diering, C. L., & Palmer, M. H. (2001). Professional information about urinary incontinence on the World Wide Web: Is it timely? Is it accurate? *The Journal of Wound, Ostomy, and Incontinence Nursing, 28*, 55–62.

Eng, T. E., Maxfield, A., Patrick, K., Deering, M. J., Ratzan, S. C., & Gustafson, D. H. (1998). Access to health information and support: A public highway or a private road? *Journal of American Medical Society, 10*, 1371–1375.

Fitzpatrick, J. J., Romano, C., & Chasek, R. (Eds.). (2001). *The nurses' guide to consumer health Web sites*. New York: Springer Publishing Co.

Flatley-Brennan, P. (1998). Computer network home care demonstration: A randomized trial in persons living with AIDS. *Computers in Biology and Medicine, 28*, 489–508.

Gillespie, G. (2000). A recipe for tomorrow's Internets. *Health Data Management, 12*, 34–44.

Gray, J. E., Safran, C., Davis, R. B., Pomilio-Weitnzer, G., Stewart, J. E., Zaccagnini, L., & Pursley, D. (2000). Baby CareLink: Using the Internet and telemedicine to improve care for high-risk infants. *Pediatrics, 106*, 1318–1324.

Griffiths, K. M., & Christensen, H. (2000). Quality of Web based information on treatment of depression: Cross sectional survey. *British Medical Journal, 321*, 1511–1515.

Harbage, B., & Dean, A. G. (1999). Distribution of Epi Info software. *American Journal of Preventative Medicine, 16*, 314–317.

Holloway, N., Kripps, B., Koepke, K., & Skiba, D. (2000). Evaluating health care information on the Internet. In J. J. Fitzpatrick & K. S. Montgomery (Eds.), *Internet resources for nurses.* New York: Springer Publishing.

Kelley, B. (2000). Intranets succumb to irresistible pull of e-health. *Health Data Management, 12*, 56–64.

Kim, H. E., Kim, E., & Kim, J. W. (2001). Development of a breast self-examination program for the Internet. *Cancer Nursing, 24*, 156–161.

Krantz, J., Ballard, J., & Scher, J. (1997). Comparing the results of laboratory and World Wide Web samples on the determinants of female attractiveness. *Behavior Research Methods, Instruments, and Computers, 29*, 264–269.

Lakeman, R. (1997). Using the Internet for data collection in nursing research. *Computers in Nursing, 15*, 269–275.

Lau, F., & Haywood, R. (2000). Building a virtual network in a community health research training program. *Journal of the American Medical Informatics Association, 7*, 361–377.

Levy, C. E., Lash, A. T., Iverson, M. A., & Dixon, R. S. (2000). Using the Internet to enable access to medical conferences. *American Journal of Physical Medicine and Rehabilitation, 79*, 509–512.

Long, C. O., Greenberg, A., Isemurt, R. L., & Smith, G. (2000). Computer and Internet use by home care and hospice agencies. *Home Healthcare Nurse, 18*, 666–671.

National Telecommunications and Information Administration. (2000). *Falling through the net: Toward digital inclusion* [on-line]. Available: http://www.ntia.doc.gov/

Rettie, R. (2001). An exploration of flow during Internet use. *Internet Research: Networking, Applications, and Policy, 11*(2), 103–113.

Schleyer, T. K. L., & Forrest, J. L. (2000). Methods for the design and administration of web-based surveys. *Journal of the American Medical Informatics Association, 7*, 416–425.

Senior, C., Phillips, M., Barnes, J., & David, A. (1999). An investigation into the perception of dominance from schematic faces: A study using the World-Wide-Web. *Behavior Research Methods, Instruments, and Computers, 31*, 341–346.

Smith, M., & Leigh, B. (1997). Virtual subjects: Using the Internet as an alternative source of subjects and research environment. *Behavior Research, Methods, Instruments, and Computers, 29*, 260–263.

Smith, M. A., & Senior, C. (2001). The Internet and clinical psychology: A general review of the implications. *Clinical Psychology Review, 21*, 129–136.

Soetikno, R. M., Mrad, R., Pao, V., & Lenert, L. A. (1997). Quality-of-life research on the Internet: Feasibility and potential biases in patients with ulcerative colitis. *Journal of the American Medical Informatics Association, 4*, 426–435.

Suarez-Almazor, M. E., Kendall, C. J., & Dorgan, M. (2001). Surfing the net—Information on the World Wide Web for persons with arthritis: Patient empowerment or patient deceit? *The Journal of Rheumatology, 28*, 185–192.

Thomas, B., Stamler, L. L., Lafreniere, K., & Dumala, R. (2000). The Internet: An effective tool for nursing research with women. *Computers in Nursing, 16*, 13–18.

Turner, J. L., & Turner, D. B. (1999). Using the Internet to perform survey research. *Syllabus, 12*, 55–56.

Wheeler, D. C., & O'Kelly, M. E. (1999). Network topology and city accessibility of the commercial Internet. *Professional Geographer, 51*, 327–339.

Wolfgram Memorial Library (1999). Checklist for an informational web page. [Online]. Available: *http://www.science.widener.edu/'withers/inform.htm*

Zhang, Y. (1999). Using the Internet for survey research: A case study. *Journal of the American Society for Information Science, 51*, 57–68.

_____ Chapter 19

Interdisciplinary Collaboration

Patricia Hinton Walker

_____

U se of the Internet for interdisciplinary purposes should be considered an evolving challenge. What is known today as "interdisciplinary or collaborative practice" actually began as early as
the 1900s when missionaries in India used interprofessional teams to
provide health services to communities. Historical notes reveal that
"After WWII, interprofessional teams were used to meet multiple needs
of the chronically ill; in the 1960's the federal government encouraged
interdisciplinary teams at neighborhood health centers; and in the
1970's and 1980's the Veterans Administration funded a nation-wide
effort to train teams for care of aging veterans" (Walker et al., 1998,
p. 88). Although there appears to be a significant historical perspective
that interdisciplinary teams are of value both clinically and economically, much of the literature highlights the challenges and barriers to
interdisciplinary education, practice, and research. The majority of the
literature supporting interdisciplinary practice and education consists
of descriptions of models of care and/or model education programs.

   Although the Internet has great potential for use in interdisciplinary
collaboration, like the history previously mentioned, the challenges still
outweigh the progress. The nursing profession has historically viewed
itself as interdisciplinary collaborators with many health care professions—medicine, social work, psychology, and pharmacy to name a
few. Most practicing nurses also would see themselves collaborating
on a daily basis to achieve improved patient care and outcomes in
hospitals, nursing homes, and home-health and other community-

based settings. In many of these cases, the nurse initiates the collaborative effort and this is also true for the use of the Internet for interdisciplinary collaboration among disciplines.

This chapter will highlight some of the possibilities and challenges for nurses who are interested in the use of the Internet for interdisciplinary collaboration. Initially, the approach will be fairly traditional by exploring what is available on the Internet related to interdisciplinary practice, education and research. Suggestions for searching the Web will be included, as well as options the author has explored, and brief summaries of information that resulted from Internet searches. Finally, creative approaches and nontraditional perspectives will be presented that may stimulate colleagues to explore new directions on the Web and use the Web in innovative and different ways related to interdisciplinary collaboration.

INTERDISCIPLINARY PRACTICE

Many of the options for use of the Internet for interdisciplinary practice would best be described as one-on-one communications between and among providers. Nurses (particularly APNs) can use the Internet to collaborate with other providers by e-mail, particularly with back-up physicians, pharmacists, and social workers. This important tool would be particularly valuable to nurses practicing in rural communities where distance may be a factor. However, one of the greatest challenges, particularly in many rural communities, is access and interest (for both providers) in use of the Internet for collaborative practice communication.

The Internet can clearly enhance interdisciplinary communication. However, many providers prefer the phone-fax combination. At this time, faxes and telephones remain the favorite method of communication of lab results and other information, frequently because of the time and effort it takes to retype the information. One barrier is the lack of systems within practice settings and other institutions that support Internet collaborative practice. For example, although e-mail may be accessible, auxiliary departments such as the lab, x-ray, and pharmacy are not even intranet connected in many health care systems. Perhaps providers who have established a longer-term personal relationship and are comfortable with different forms of communication could use the Internet more easily. An important challenge in this area is the concern for patient confidentiality, and there may also be other legal risks to consider related to electronic consultation and the way this is documented. (Please see chapter 9 for additional information on security issues related to using the Internet in patient care settings.)

When searching the Web for possibilities related to interdisciplinary practice, the author discovered that the word "health" must be inserted into the search. The key word "interdisciplinary health practice" provided several interesting results. First, federal agencies that are interested in interdisciplinary practice surfaced. One of the most important agencies was the Institute of Medicine (IOM).

"The mission of the Institute of Medicine is to advance and disseminate scientific knowledge to improve human health. The Institute provides objective, timely, authoritative information and advice concerning health and science policy to government, the corporate sector, the professions and the public" (Institute of Medicine Web site, 2001). This Web site (*www4.nationalacademies.org/iom/iomhome.nsf*) provides information related to activities, programs, and reports of the IOM, which are of interest for interdisciplinary practice. Many of the activities address global and international issues, but of interest to health care providers from all disciplines are recent programs and publications. Copies of important IOM reports such as "Crossing the Quality Chasm: A New Health System for the 21st Century," "Improving the Quality of Long-Term Care," and "Protecting Data Privacy in Health Services Research" are available online and should be of particular interest to nurses considering the implications of improving quality of care through interdisciplinary collaboration.

Another agency that encourages and supports interdisciplinary practice is the National Academies of Practice (NAP). Their Web site (*http://views.vcu.edu/nap/memberinfo.htm*) mission statement indicates areas of focus. The NAP is an organization devoted to "promoting quality health care for all through interdisciplinary practice, education and research" (NAP Web site, 2001). Members of the NAP represent the following professions: dentistry, medicine, nursing, optometry, osteopathic medicine, pharmacy, podiatry, psychology, social work, and veterinary medicine. Recently the NAP has added a journal devoted to interdisciplinary care, *The National Academies of Practice Forum* (NAP Web site, 2001).

Problem areas in health care that are truly interdisciplinary in nature also are related to interdisciplinary practice. One such issue that has recently received a great deal of press coverage is the issue of medication errors and other aspects of patient safety. One important site addressing this issue is the National Patient Safety Foundation (NPSF) (*www.npsf.org/*) whose mission is "to improve measurable patient safety in the delivery of health care by its efforts to: identify and create a core body of knowledge; identify pathways to apply the knowledge; develop and enhance the culture of receptivity to patient safety; raise public awareness and foster communications about patient safety" (National Patient Safety Foundation Web site, 2001). Web sites such as this one provide bibliographic resources and focus on medication errors and many other patient safety factors that have been historically of interest to nurses, but are an interdisciplinary issue. There is ample opportunity for nurses to contact these sites and begin a dialogue with others in chat rooms. It will be important for nurses to interact with other disciplines in order for nursing perspectives to be highlighted and included in the multidisciplinary approaches to addressing clinical problems.

Finally, a recently published book by the editors of this book, *Internet Resources for Nurses* (Fitzpatrick & Montgomery, 2000) provides nurses with a wealth of Internet resources related to specific diseases and/or conditions. A number of Web sites identified and evaluated in this book are important linkages for interdisciplinary practice. Good examples are presented in the chapters on pharmaceutical resources, HIV/AIDS, cancer, and advanced practice. The chapter on pharmaceutical resources provides excellent resources for APNs who are prescribing, such as Medical World Search (*www.mwsearch.com*) and RxMed (*www.rxmed.com*). These sites provide information related to pharmaceutical products and are an excellent interdisciplinary resource for practicing nurses.

Two other chapters are examples of how nurses may use interdisciplinary sites for practice. The chapters on HIV/AIDS and cancer have a number of sites that would serve as resources to determine latest treatment options, downloading of reports (research and statistics) and information related to the latest clinical trials. In addition to some of the most well known sites such as the Centers for Disease Control and Prevention (*www.cdc.gov*) and the American Cancer Society (*www.cancer.org*), this new book evaluates a number of other sites that would be of interest to nurses for patient care, patient advocacy, and/or participation in treatment (Fitzpatrick & Montgomery, 2000).

Last of all, Internet sites are evaluated for all types of symptom management, many developed by other disciplines. In the Fitzpatrick and Montgomery (2000) book one additional site is important to mention as an example here: MD Consult (*www.mdconsult.com*) is a fee-based site where APNs can obtain physician consultation for practice. However, two other sites should be mentioned: *The Merck Manual* (*www.merck.com/pubs/mmanual*) is a "virtual" medical textbook that is used by health care providers worldwide as an important reference, and the National Guideline Clearinghouse Web page (*www.guideline.gov/body_home.asp*) is an important resource for evidence-based practice that is produced by the Agency for Healthcare Research and Quality (AHRQ) in collaboration with the American Medical Association (AMA) and the American Association of Health Plans (AAHP) (Fitzpatrick & Montgomery, 2000). Many APNs now practice in managed care settings, consequently guidelines for evidence-based practice in collaboration with physicians in the system in becoming increasingly important.

INTERDISCIPLINARY EDUCATION

The following sites can be very helpful to nurses who are interested in learning more or teaching interdisciplinary education. Medscape (*www.medscape.com*) provides free full-text access to recent clinical topics, and use of Virtual Hospital (*www.vh.org/Providers/Simulations/PatientSimulations.html*) is a great resource for teaching interdisciplinary groups because of case studies and teaching tools related to hospital care (Fitzpatrick & Montgomery, 2000). These two examples of general Web sites are excellent resources for interdisciplinary education since access to recent publications and presentations are free, along with other information, multimedia resources, case studies, and teaching tools.

Interdisciplinary education is an important priority of the Association of Academic Health Centers (AHC). The mission and purpose of this organization is stated on their Web site (*www.ahcnet.org/*), i.e., "to improve the health of the people by advancing the leadership of academic health centers in health professions education, biomedical and health services research, and health care delivery" (AHC Web site, 2001). With more than 100 institutions responsible for education in the health professions, biomedical and health services research, and many aspects of patient care as members, this association also has a commitment to interdisciplinary education. The topic "Cross-Professions" on the AHC Web site provides information on innovative and noteworthy models of interdisciplinary education and practice at academic health centers nationwide (AHC Web site, 2001).

Highlighted under "Cross-Professions" on the Web site is The Center for Interdisciplinary, Community-Based Learning (CICL). Established in January 1997 as a cooperative agreement between the Association of Academic Health Centers (AHC) and the U.S. Department of Health and Human Services, the CICL's primary objectives are to:

- Strengthen and institutionalize academic health centers' commitment to interdisciplinary, community-based learning, particularly in underserved areas
- Provide expertise to academic health centers with respect to model curricula, training sites, and relationships with community care facilities for interdisciplinary, community-based learning
- Support an interdisciplinary network of health care professionals who are working to create and strengthen an interdisciplinary, community-based curriculum (AHC Web site, 2001)

There is an extensive CICL annotated bibliography available free of charge for those interested in interdisciplinary education. The majority of the topics in the bibliography are focused on interdisciplinary education, with some publications on practice and research.

An annotated bibliography (located at *http://www.uth.tmc.edu/sacs/ bib.html*) is very complete and has numerous references related to success stories and challenges of interdisciplinary education and practice. Of the 198 publications, slightly over 1/3 (36%) of the articles are authored by nurses or related to the nursing profession. In addition to the references related to education, this annotated bibliography describes numerous publications related to interdisciplinary practice and research as well. As mentioned previously, much of the literature and resources available in this area deals with demonstration projects or models at different settings and universities.

Finally, it is important to consider the use of chat rooms and sites that provide for online discussion. One such site is Leading Organizations to Health, consisting of "a community of leaders who are passionate about creating healthy and vital organizations" (Leading Organizations to Health Web site, 2001). This group (whose e-mail address is *lead-org-health@yahoogroups.com*) features open discussion among leaders and colleagues on addressing workplace challenges by creating work environments that call forth creativity, collaboration, active engagement, and commitment in their people. This site provides opportunities for discussion with different disciplines related to health care practice, policy, and organizational issues.

Blackboard (*www.blackboard.com*) and Education World (*www.education-world.com*) are Internet resources that should be mentioned because they provide faculty members with opportunities to place course outlines and teaching materials online. These sites are helpful when the challenges of different platforms and/or systems are used and/or not available to all disciplines involved in the interdisciplinary education effort. Both of these programs facilitate interaction between the faculty and students and, more important, among students from different disciplines.

INTERDISCIPLINARY RESEARCH

Even more challenging for Internet exploration is the topic of interdisciplinary research. Results of interdisciplinary research are published, but there is a dearth of publications specifically on interdisciplinary research. This is also true when searching the Internet. Besides the two bibliographies previously mentioned which contained publications related to interdisciplinary research, there is little available. Consequently, using the Internet for online exploration of interdisciplinary collaboration takes nurses to some governmental sites that support interdisciplinary research and facilitate interdisciplinary research funding, presentations, and publications through their organizations.

The first and most obvious place to explore the potential for interdisciplinary research is the National Institutes of Health (*www.nih.gov*). The NIH, one of eight health agencies of the Public Health Service is part of the U.S. Department of Health and Human Services. The NIH mission is "to uncover new knowledge that will lead to better health for everyone." NIH works toward that mission by: conducting research in its own laboratories; supporting the research of non-Federal scientists in universities, medical schools, hospitals, and research institutions throughout the country and abroad; helping in the training of research investigators; and fostering communication of medical information. There are 27 separate institutes and centers, many of which are of interest to nurses and the nursing profession, and many of these welcome interdisciplinary research of which nurses may participate such as: aging, child health and human development, and the cancer institute.

Another governmental site is the Agency for Healthcare Research and Quality (AHRQ) (*www.ahrq.gov*), which "provides evidence-based information on health care outcomes, quality and cost, use, and access. Information from AHRQ's research helps people make more informed decisions and improve the quality of health care services" (Agency for Healthcare Research and Quality Web site, 2001). The Academy for Health Services Research (*www.ahsrhp.org/*) may also be a useful resource. "In June 2000, the Alpha Center and the Association for Health Services Research merged to form the Academy for Health Services Research and Health Policy. The Academy provides a professional home and technical assistance resource for researchers and policy professionals. Committed to the vision of improving health and health care by generating new knowledge and moving knowledge into action, the Academy seeks to stimulate the development, understanding, and use of the best available health services research and health policy information by public and private decision makers" (Academy for Health Services Research Web site, 2001).

Behavioral research is another type of interdisciplinary research. One site, the Center for Advancement of Health (CFAH), would be of particular interest to nurses whose research focus is related to behavioral change. According to the CFAH Web site (*www.cfah.org/*) "Biobehavioral research examines the links among biology, behavior, psychology, and social context. Its findings add to our understanding of the mechanisms of disease onset and progression, effective health promotion, and disease prevention strategies, and interventions that help people with chronic diseases to more successfully manage their conditions. . . . The Center for the Advancement of Health seeks to close this gap between evidence to practice by: strengthening the capacity of the biobehavioral research community to conduct high-quality research; communicating research findings to decision-makers and the public; translating and integrating research findings into the real world of health care policy and practice" (CFAH Web site, 2001).

Again, it is important to note that this area is a particular challenge for Internet use. However, nurses should become more active in participation with other disciplines in research and engage in discussions with members of other disciplines on these Web sites whenever and wherever possible. One of the challenges for nurses is to make the nursing profession and the results of nursing research more visible to other disciplines. Also, there is great potential for the use of Federal and nonprofit databases by nurses, along with other disciplines. Use by nurses may begin to highlight the relevance of the data to nursing and the relevance of nursing to the data used and collected by other researchers. Finally, there is great potential for interdisciplinary collaboration between and among researchers by just using e-mail, searches, sharing of data, and chat rooms. This is not a common approach at this time and there is very little in the literature about use of the Internet for interdisciplinary research.

CREATIVE USE OF THE INTERNET TO STRENGTHEN NURSING'S COLLABORATIVE EFFORTS

In this chapter the author has focused on many of the challenges in, and has provided general resources that would be helpful for, interdisciplinary collaboration. Although this is an underdeveloped area, it is important to remember that the Internet provides many opportunities for nurses to be more informed when communicating (whether in person or on the Internet) with practitioners in other disciplines. Information that has previously been primarily accessible only to another discipline (except when reviewing literature in the library) is now much more accessible on the Web. For example, take the case of collaboration with pharmacists. There is a tremendous amount of information on the Web related to pharmaceutical products and treatment of conditions and diseases. Nurses, armed with information from the Internet can be more confident and participate more fully as patient/client advocates in discussions of treatment options, including medications.

However, there is also an important opportunity for interdisciplinary collaboration beyond the traditional disciplines with which nurses usually collaborate. The Internet has opened the door in significant ways for the use of alternative approaches to care. Although the consumer (even health care providers) should be careful in reviewing data related to alternative approaches, frequently patients/clients seek new and different approaches to care such as music therapy, use of herbs and other natural products, relaxation therapy, and all forms of touch therapies to replace and/or enhance traditional health care treatment. Results from a 1997 survey indicated that 43% of an estimated 40.6 million adults in the U.S. accessed the Internet to obtain health care information (Ferguson, 1998). There are a number of Web sites that provide information related to alternative and complementary medicine including Alternative Health News Online (*www.altmedicine.com*) which has an extensive search engine for specific topics, and The National Center for Complementary and Alternative Medicine (*www.nccam.nih.gov*) which provides research-based information and a clearinghouse (Fitzpatrick & Montgomery, 2000). There are also alternative and complementary medicine sites for specific conditions such as asthma, stroke, and women's health. In addition, a number of universities have Web sites and provide information related to alternative/complementary health care.

Another organization that is committed to bringing individuals together across disciplines is the Association of Healing Health Care Projects (AHHCP). This organization "commits to creating an intentional future for health care based on the ethic of health ourselves, our relationships, and our communities, and brings together individuals and organizations whose interest and involvement include the allopathic medical model, alternative/complementary practices, and relationship-centered care" (Association of Healing Health Care Projects Web site, 2001). This is a "virtual organization" which remains inclusive of all who elect to embrace its philosophy and objectives.

Finally, other nontraditional sites may be of interest to nurses who are searching on specific topics such as pain management and/or symptom management, for example, *www.medicalresonancetherapymusic.com* and *www.scientificmusictherapy.com*. In the nursing literature, music and other alternative therapies have been the topic of research for symptom management; consequently nontraditional sites such as these may be of interest. Consumers are very interested in alternative/complementary therapies and are using the Internet to explore options for care. This is an emerging area where the nursing profession can link with other disciplines that are focused on holistic care.

Several private foundations have demonstrated interest in interdisciplinary education, practice, and research through their funding priorities. Following are three examples of foundations supporting interdisciplinary education. The Fetzer Institute (*www.fetzer.org/*) focuses on integral relationships among body, mind, and spirit. Other areas supported by the Fetzer Institute are relationship-centered care and leadership development (Fetzer Institute Web site, 2001). The Pew Charitable Trusts (*www.pewtrusts.com*) health and human service programs are "designed to promote the health and well being of the American people and to strengthen disadvantaged communities" (Pew Charitable Trusts Web site, 2001). Finally, the John A. Hartford Foundation (*www.jhartfound.org/*) is "a committed champion of health care training, research, and service system innovations that will ensure the well-being and vitality of older adults" (John A. Hartford Foundation Web site, 2001). These foundations continue to provide opportunities for grant funding to support innovative, interdisciplinary projects, and are potential resources that nurses should use for financial support of new interdisciplinary projects.

Nurses are frequently the first source of information for patients and are usually responsible for much of the patient education that is documented. Faced with consumer interest and access to new health care information on the Internet, nurses will be increasingly challenged to respond to patients regarding interdisciplinary information available on the Internet. Again, by taking the initiative, nurses can use the Internet wisely to improve communication both with patients and with other disciplines.

CONCLUSIONS

Although this chapter focuses on many of the challenges of Internet use, it is important to for nurses to think about practical ways of using the Internet for interdisciplinary collaboration. Armed with better information regarding the latest decisions, pharmaceuticals, and treatment options from the Internet, nurses can be stronger advocates for their patients/ clients. Also, by working with patients and clients who will search the Internet for information regarding their diseases/conditions and treatment options, nurses can interface with other disciplines more effectively.

The nursing profession will continue to provide health care in a collaborative manner. However, astute nurses will use the Internet to explore up-to-date options and become more knowledgeable about content that used to be "privileged information" for one discipline or another. The Internet has the potential to "empower" both the nurse and the patient/client in communicating and working collaboratively with other disciplines. As professionals, nurses must see themselves as "empowered" to explore the Internet for answers and ammunition for discussions, debates, and patient advocacy issues. Although a more informed nurse armed with the latest information may make interdisciplinary colleagues uncomfortable at times, the Internet provides the nursing profession with the opportunity to enhance the patient/client advocacy role (one of our historical strengths) and make it central to our practice.

Students in educational programs should also be encouraged to use the Internet to explore both advances in nursing care, as well as advances in treatment options for their patients. Nurses can assist patient/clients in their decision making by making sure that they are informed of the latest options, risks, and effectiveness of different treatment plans. However, we also have significant challenges within the profession to encourage nurses at all levels to explore the Internet in education, practice, and research. Like other health care professionals, nurses need to overcome some of the historical barriers to the use of technology and explore ways to balance the use of technology with the science of caring. Both are critical to improved outcomes and satisfaction in the 21st century.

WEB SITE RECAP

Academy for Health Services Research
http://www.ahsrhp.org/

Agency for Healthcare Research and Quality
http://www.ahrq.gov

Alternative Health News Online
http://www.altmedicine.com

American Cancer Society
http://www.cancer.org

Association of Academic Health Centers
http://www.ahcnet.org/

Blackboard
http://www.blackboard.com

Center for Advancement of Health
http://www.cfah.org/

Centers for Disease Control and Prevention
http://www.cdc.gov

Education World
http://www.education-world.com

The Fetzer Institute
http://www.fetzer.org/

Institute of Medicine
http://www4.nationalacademics.org/iom/iomhome.nsf

John A. Hartford Foundation
http://www.jhartfound.org/

Leading Organizations to Health
http://lead-org-health@yahoogroups.com

MD Consult
http://www.mdconsult.com

Medical Resonance Therapy Music
http://www.medicalresonancetherapymusic.com

Medical World Search
http://www.mwsearch.com

Medscape
http://www.medscape.com

The Merck Manual
http://www.merck.com/pubs/mmanual

National Academies of Practice
http://views.vcu.edu/nap/memberinfo.htm

The National Center for Complementary and Alternative Medicine
http://www.nccam.nih.gov

National Guideline Clearinghouse
http://www.guideline.gov/body_home.asp

National Institutes of Health
http://www.nih.gov

National Patient Safety Foundation
http://www.npsf.org/

The Pew Charitable Trusts
http://www.pewtrusts.com

RxMed
http://www.rxmed.com

Scientific Music Therapy
http://www.scientificmusictherapy.com

University of Texas Health Sciences Center at Houston's Annotated Bibliography of Articles on Interdisciplinary or Related Subjects
http://www.uth.tmc.edu/sacs.bib.html

Virtual Hospital: Patient Simulations
http://www.vh.org/Providers/Simulations/PatientSimulations.html

REFERENCES

Academy for Health Services Research (2001). [Online]. Available: *http://www. ahsrhp.org/*.

Agency for Healthcare Research and Quality (2001). [Online]. Available: *http:// www.ahrq.gov*.

Association of Academic Health Centers (2001). [Online]. Available: *www.ahcnet. org/*.

Association of Healing Health Care Projects (2001). [Online]. Available: *http:// www.healinghealthcareassoc.org/*.

Center for Advancement of Health (2001). [Online]. Available: *http://www.cfah.org/*.

Ferguson, T. (1998). Digital doctoring—opportunities and challenges in electronic patient-physician communication (editorial). *The Journal of the American Medical Association, 280*, 1361–1362.

Fetzer Institute. (2001). [Online]. Available: *http://www.fetzer.org/*.

Fitzpatrick, J. J., & Montgomery, K. S. (Eds.). (2000). *Internet resources for nurses.* New York: Springer Publishing Co.

Institute of Medicine. (2001). [Online]. Available: *http://www4/nationalacademies.org/iom/iomhome.nsf*.

John A. Hartford Foundation. (2001). [Online]. Available: *http://www.jhartround.org/*.

Leading Organizations to Health. (2001). [Online]. Available: *lead-org-health@yahoogroups.com*.

National Academies of Practice. (2001). [Online]. Available: *http://views.vcu.edu/nap/memberinfo/html*.

National Patient Safety Foundation. (2001). [Online]. Available: *http://www.npsf.org/*.

Pew Charitable Trusts. (2001). [Online]. Available: *http://www.pewtrusts.com*.

Walker, P. H., Baldwin, D., Fitzpatrick, J. J., Ryan, S., Bulger, R., DeBasio, N., Hanson, C., Harvan, R., Johnson-Pawlson, J., Kelley, M., Lacey, B., Ladden, M. J., McLaughlin, C., Selker, L., Sluyter, D., & Vanselow, N. (1998). Building community: Developing skills for interprofessional health. *Nursing Outlook, 46*, 88–89.

Appendix

ALPHABETICAL INDEX OF WEB SITES LISTED

Web Site	Section	Page number
American Academy of Nurse Practitioners *http://www.aanp.org*	Health care policy and legal issues	208, 213
American Association of Critical Care Nurses *http://www.aacn.org*	Nursing staff recruitment; Continuing education	77, 80
American Cancer Society *http://www.cancer.org*	Interdisciplinary collaboration	232, 240
American Dietetics Association *http://www.eatright.org*	Classroom	186, 191
Amorican Nurses Association *http://www.ana.org*	Health care policy and legal issues	208, 213
American Nurses Association Capitol Wiz *http://www.nursingworld.org/ gova/state_v1.htm*	APN issues	165, 168
Ask Jeeves *http://www.ask.com*	Skill building and practice	36, 44
Association for periOperative Registered Nurses *http://www.aorn.org*	Nursing staff recruitment; Continuing education	77, 81, 195, 200
Association of Academic Health Centers *http://www.ahcnet.org/*	Interdisciplinary collaboration	233, 240
Association of Women's Health, Obstetrics, and Neonatal Nurses *http://www.awhonn.org*	Continuing education	195, 200
Auscultation Assistant at UCLA *http://www.wilkes.med.ucla.edu/ intro.html*	APN issues	160, 168

Web Site	Section	Page number
Blackboard *http://www.blackboard.com*	Interdisciplinary collaboration	235, 240
Bob Bowman's Educational Technologies *http://www.user.shentel.net/ rbowman/.*	Using the Internet in clinical settings	23
Careermosaic.com *http://www.careermosaic.com*	Nursing staff recruitment	77, 81
Center for Advancement of Health *http://www.cfah.org/*	Interdisciplinary collaboration	236, 240
Centers for Disease Control and Prevention *http://www.cdc.gov*	Staff development; Research; Interdisciplinary collaboration	68, 221, 226, 232, 240
Central Nervous System Infection Cases *http://edcenter.med.cornell.edu/ Pathophysiology_Cases/CNS/ CNS_TOCs.html*	Skill building and practice	38, 44
Commission on Accreditation of Rehabilitation Facilities *http://www.carf.org*	Improving performance	54, 60
Common Questions About Integrating the Internet into the Classroom *http://www.iloveteaching.com/ Intenetclass/index.htm*	Classroom	190, 192
Concept Media *http://www.conceptmedia.com*	Skill building and practice	38, 44
Congressional Record Text *http://thomas.loc.gov/*	Health care policy and legal issues	209, 213
Cumulative Index of Nursing and Allied Health Literature (CINAHL) *http://www.cinahl.com*	Staff development; APN issues	68, 163, 168

Web Site	Section	Page number
Delaware Academy of Medicine *http://www.delamed.org/ chlsweblinks.html*	APN issues	167, 168
Delightinceptions.com *http://www.delightinceptions.com*	Nursing staff recruitment	70, 81
Digiscript *http://library.digiscript.com*	Staff development	67, 68
The Dermatology Internet Service *http://www.dermis.net*	Skill building and practice	38, 45
Education World *http://www.education-world.com*	Interdisciplinary collaboration	235, 241
e-Medtools *http://www.e-medtools.com*	APN issues	165, 168
Epocrates *http://www.epocrates.com*	APN issues	165, 168
Eye Simulator *http://cim.ucdavis.edu/eyes/ eyesim.htm*	Skill building and practice; APN issues	38, 44, 160, 168
Federal Register *http://www.access.gpo.gov/ su_docs/aces/aces140.html*	Health care policy and legal issues	209, 213
The Fetzer Institute *http://www.fetzer.org*	Interdisciplinary collaboration	238, 241
Firewalls *http://www.vicomsoft.com/ knowledge/reference/ firewalls1.html?track=internal*	Security concerns	114, 116
Foodfit.com *http://www.foodfit.com*	Classroom	186, 192
Google *http://www.google.com*	Skill building and practice	36, 44
HandheldMed *http://www.handheldmed.com*	APN issues	165, 168

Web Site	Section	Page number
John A. Hartford Foundation *http://www.jhartfound.org/*	Interdisciplinary collaboration	239, 241
Headhunter.net *http://www.headhunter.net*	Nursing staff recruitment	77, 81
Health on the Net (HON) Foundation Code of Conduct *http://www.hon.ch/HONcode/Conduct.html*	Accessing current research and practice information; Skill building and practice	5, 10, 44
Health Stream E-Learning *http://www.healthstream.com*	Staff development	67, 68
Healthfinder *http://www.healthfinder.gov*	APN issues	162, 169
Information Quality World Wide Web Virtual Library *http://www.ciolek.com/WWWVL-InfoQuality.html*	Health care policy and legal issues	211, 213
Ingenta *http://www.ingenta.com*	Accessing current research and practice information	6, 10
Inner Body *http://www.innerbody.com/htm/anim.html*	Skill building and practice	38, 44
Institute of Medicine *http:// www4.nationalacademies.org/iom/iomhome.nsf*	Interdisciplinary collaboration	231, 241
Interactive Crash Cart *http://web.ucdmc.ucdavis.edu/edu/Resources/Resources.htm*	Staff development	68
Internet Activities for Foreign Language Classes *http://members.aol.com/maestro12/web/wadir.html*	Classroom	189, 192

Web Site	Section	Page number
Internet Business Network *http://www.interbiznet.com*	Nursing staff recruitment	81
Internet in the Classroom: First Steps *http://home.swbell.net/jraneri/ internetintheclassroom.htm*	Classroom	190, 192
Joint Commission on Accreditation of Health Care Organizations *http://www.jcaho.org*	Staff development; Improving performance	54, 60, 62, 69
The Journal of Continuing Education in Nursing *http://www.slackinc.com/allied/ jcen/jcenhome.htm*	Continuing education	198, 200
Leading Organizations to Health *http://lead-org-health@yahoogroups.com*	Interdisciplinary collaboration	234, 241, 242
Learn the Net *http://www.learnthenet.com*	Skill building and practice	36, 44
MD Consult *http://www.mdconsult.com*	Interdisciplinary collaboration	233, 241
Medical Resonance Therapy Music *http://www. medicalresonancetherapymusic.com*	Interdisciplinary collaboration	238, 241
Medical World Search *http://www.mwsearch.com*	Interdisciplinary collaboration	232, 241
Medimorphus.com *http://www.medimorphus.com*	Nursing staff recruitment	81
MEDLINE/PubMed *http://www.ncbi.nlm.nih.gov/ entrez/query.fcgi*	APN issues	163, 169

Web Site	Section	Page number
MEDLINEplus at the National Library of Medicine *http://www.medlineplus.gov/*	APN issues	162, 169
Medscape *http://www.medscape.com*	Interdisciplinary collaboration	233, 241
Medsite *http://www.medsite.com*	Skill building and practice	38, 44
The Merck Manual *http://www.merck.com/pubs/ mmanual*	Interdisciplinary collaboration	233, 241
Monster Jobs *http://www.monster.com*	Nursing staff recruitment	77, 81
National Academies of Practice *http://views.vcu.edu/nap/ memberinfo.htm*	Interdisciplinary collaboration	231, 241
The National Center for Complementary and Alternative Medicine *http://www.nccam.nih.gov*	Interdisciplinary collaboration	238, 241
National Guideline Clearinghouse *http://www.guideline.gov/ body_home.asp*	Accessing current research and practice information; Improving performance; Staff development; Interdisciplinary collaboration	7, 10, 52, 60, 65, 233, 241
National Institutes of Health *http://www.nih.gov*	Interdisciplinary collaboration	235, 241
National Library of Medicine *http://www.nlm.nih.gov*	Using the Internet in clinical settings	19, 32
National Patient Safety Foundation *http://www.npsf.org/*	Interdisciplinary collaboration	232, 241
Net Learning *http://www.net-learning.com*	Staff development	68, 69
Netiquette *http://www.albion.com/ netiquette/book/index.html*	Using the Internet in clinical settings	29, 33

Web Site	Section	Page number
Neurological Examination *http://www.medinfo.ufl.edu/ year1/bcs/clist/neuro.html*	Skill building and practice	38, 44
North American Nursing Diagnosis Association *http://www.nanda.org*	Skill building and practice	39, 44
Nurse CEU *http://www.nurseceu.com/*	Using the Internet in clinical settings	33
Nurse Learn *http://www.nurselearn.com/ free_online_training.htm*	Skill building and practice	38, 44
NURSENET *http:// www.graduateresearch.com/ NurseNet*	Skill building and practice	38, 44
NurseWeek *http://www.nurseweek.com/*	Using the Internet in clinical settings; Nursing staff recruitment	33, 78, 81
Nursing Interventions Classification *http://www.nursing.uiowa.edu/nic*	Skill building and practice	39, 44
Nursing Outcomes Classification *http://www.nursing.uiowa.edu/ noc/index.htm*	Skill building and practice	39, 45
Nursing Spectrum *http://www.nursingspectrum.com*	Nursing staff recruitment	78, 81
Nursingcenter.com *http://www.nursingcenter.com*	APN issues	164, 169
Nursinghands.com *http://www.nursinghands.com*	Nursing staff recruitment	78, 81
NYU Patient and Family Resource Center *http://library.med.nyu.edu/HCC/*	Accessing current research and practice information	5, 10

Web Site	Section	Page number
Occupational Safety and Health Administration *http://www.osha.gov*	Staff development	69
Oncolink at the University of Pennsylvania *http://cancer.med.upenn.edu*	APN issues	162, 169
PDA Cortex *http://www.rnpalm.com*	APN issues	165, 169
Peterson's-Distance Learning *http://www.lifelonglearning.com*	Undergraduate education	138
The Pew Charitable Trusts *http://www.pewtrusts.com*	Interdisciplinary collaboration	238
Physicians' Desk Reference Online *http://www.pdr.net/*	APN issues	169
Quack Watch *http://www.quackwatch.com*	Skill building and practice	43, 45
QwestDex *http://www.qwestdex.com/*	Using the Internet in clinical settings	30, 33
The R.A.L.E. Repository *http://www.rale.ca*	APN issues	160, 169
Resources for Reducing Medication Errors and Improving Quality in Hospitals *http://www.mederror.com*	Staff development	69
RxMed *http://www.rxmed.com*	Interdisciplinary collaboration	232, 242
Scientific Music Therapy *http:// www.scientificmusictherapy.com*	Interdisciplinary collaboration	238, 242

Web Site	Section	Page number
Sigma Theta Tau International *http://www.nursingsociety.org*	Improving performance	52, 60
Springer Publishing Company *http://www.springerpub.com*	APN issues	169
Springnet *http://www.springnet.com*	Nursing staff recruitment	77, 81
Thinking Critically about World Wide Web Resources *http://www.library.ucla.edu/ libraries/college/help/critical/ index.htm*	Skill building and practice	43, 45
37.com *http://www.37.com*	Skill building and practice	36, 43
University at Albany Libraries Evaluating Internet Resources *http://library.albany.edu/internet/ evaluate.html*	Health care policy and legal issues	211, 213
University Hospital Consortium *http://www.radsci.ucla.edu:8000/ frames/physician/uhc/index.html*	Using the Internet in clinical settings	31, 33
University of California at San Francisco Nurseweb *http://nurseweb.ucsf.edu/www/ arwwebpg.htm*	APN issues	159, 169
University of Florida Health Sciences Library *http://www.library.health.ufl.edu/ pubmed/pubmed2/overview.html*	Accessing current research and practice information	5, 10
University of Kansas Clinical Orientation Page *http://169.147.169.238/ comanual/*	Using the Internet in clinical settings	23, 33

Web Site	Section	Page number
University of Kansas Medical Center: Virtual Classroom *http://www.kumc.edu/vc*	Skill building and practice	37, 45
University of Maryland School of Nursing *http://nursing.umaryland.edu*	Skill building and practice	37, 45
University of Texas Health Sciences Center at Houston's Annotated Bibliography of Articles on Interdisciplinary or Related Subjects *http://www.uth.tmc.edu/sacs/ bib.html*	Interdisciplinary collaboration	234, 242
The U.S. Congress *http://www.congress.gov*	Health care policy and legal issues	209, 213
U.S. General Accounting Office (GAO) *http://www.gao.gov*	Health care policy and legal issues	210, 213
Using the Internet in the Classroom *http://mason.gmu.edu/ ~montecin/IDOweb-w.htm*	Classroom	190, 192
Virginia Henderson International Nursing Library *http://www.stti.iupui.edu/library/ index.html*	APN issues	163, 169
Virtual Economy Home Page *http://www.bized.ac.uk/virtual/ economy/*	Skill building and practice	39, 45
Virtual Hospital: Patient Simulations *http://www.vh.org/Providers/ Simulations/ PatientSimulations.html*	Skill building and practice; Interdisciplinary collaboration; APN issues	37, 45, 159, 169, 233, 242

Web Site	Section	Page number
Virtual Naval Hospital *http://www.vnh.org*	APN issues	159, 169
The Visible Human Project *http://www.nlm.nih.gov/research/* *visible/visible_human.html*	Skill building and practice	39, 45
The Washington Post *http://www.washingtonpost.com*	Health care policy and legal issues	209, 213
Web-CEU *http://www.webceu.com/*	Using the Internet in clinical settings	25, 33
World Health Organization (WHO) *http://www.who.org*	Research	221, 226
World Lecture Hall *http://www.utexas.edu/world/* *lecture*	Undergraduate education	138, 139
World Sarcoidosis Society *http://www.worldsarcsociety.com*	Using the Internet in clinical settings	21, 33
Yahoo! *http://www.yahoo.com*	Skill building and practice	35, 45
Yahoo!'s Pharmaceutical Company List *http://cf.us.biz.yahoo.com/p/* *_health-majrrx.html*	Using the Internet in clinical settings	20, 33
Your Internet Guides: Internet Primer *http://www.thirteen.org/edonline/* *primer*	Classroom	190, 192

Index

Springer Publishing Company

Telecommunications for Nurses
Providing Successful Distance Education and Telehealth, Second Edition

Myrna L. Armstrong, EdD, RN, FAAN,
and **Shari Frueh,** BSN, RN, Editors

"It is a book which describes how creative people, often taking a fresh approach, can get the best out of what modern distance communications technology has to offer."
—From the Foreword by **Susan M. Sparks**, RN, PhD, FAAN
Senior Education Specialist, National Library of Medicine

Totally updated and revised, this book reflects the latest developments in both distance education and telehealth, focusing on practical strategies nurses can put to use in the classroom or clinic. Each chapter is written by acknowledged experts for the particular topic. The previous edition won an American Journal of Nursing Book-of-the-Year Award.

2002   264pp   0-8261-9843-0   hard

536 Broadway, New York, NY 10012 • Telephone: 212-431-4370
Fax: 212-941-7842 • Order Toll-Free: 877-687-7476
Order On-line: www.springerpub.com

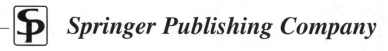

Springer Publishing Company

Distance Education in Nursing

Jeanne Novotny, PhD, RN, Editor

A comprehensive "how to" guide for designing, planning, and implementing a distance education program in your school of nursing. The emphasis is on web and Internet-Based programs. Pioneers in this fast-emerging field share their experiences with readers -- both the ups and downs. These include nurses from the University of Colorado, University of Phoenix, the Frontier School of Midwifery and Vanderbilt University. The book is appropriate for nurse educators teaching undergraduate, graduate, advanced practice, and RN students.

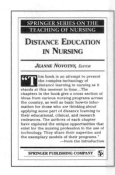

Contents:

- Distance Education Foundations, *J. M. Lewis*
- Teaching a Web-Based Course: Lessons from the Front, *M. L. McHugh and R. Gibson*
- Software Tools for Web Course Development, *R. Gibson and M. L. McHugh*
- Clinical Applications of Electronic Learning Systems, *S. M. Moore and S. J. Kelley*
- Focus on the Learner, *C. L. Mueller and D. M. Billings*
- Assessing Distance Education Programs in Nursing, *K. L. Cobb and D. M. Billings*
- Promoting Informatics in the Nursing Curriculum, *L. L. Travis*
- Distance Education at the University of Phoenix, *J. Zerwekh and S. W. Pepicello*
- Distance Graduate Education: The University of Colorado Experience,
J. K. Magilvy and M. C. Smith
- Nurse Practitioner Education: The Virginia Experience, *J. C. Novak and C. A. Corbett*
- Distance Education at the Frontier School of Midwifery and
Family Nursing: From Midwives on Horseback to Midwives on the Web,
S. E. Stone, E. K. Ernst, and S. D. Schaffer
- Supervision of RN Distance Learning Students: The Experience of
Vanderbilt's RN Bridge Program, *C. J. Bess*
- A Model for Development of a Web-Based Trauma Course, *J. E. King,*
J. Murley, S. A. Hutchison, J. Sweeney, and J. M. Novotny
- The Future of Nursing Education: Marketability, Flexibility, and Innovation, *P. H. Walker*

AJN Book of the Year Award
2000   280pp   0-8261-1341-9   hard

536 Broadway, New York, NY 10012 • Telephone: 212-431-4370
Fax: 212-941-7842 • Order Toll-Free: 877-687-7476
Order On-line: www.springerpub.com

DEMCO